Ac

Deep Water Dream

Our Indigenous community, the Teme-Augama Anishnabai (the Deep Water by the Shore People), have lived on n'Dakimenan (Our Land) for thousands of years governed by Nature's cosmic framework, 'Kou-Chee Ma-Nid-Doo (The Great Mystery). Gretchen's book provides an insider's perspective on how we, the Teme-Augama Anishnabai, began our journey of decolonization. The Cree Statesmen of the James Bay Watershed, Andy Rickard on the West side and Billy Diamond on the East side, helped us get off the ground. Jim and Gretchen's move to Bear Island, Lake Temagami, was essential for us to keep going.

— *Chief Gary Potts, Teme-Augama Anishnabai*

Deep Water Dream is a personal account of a devoted and determined family physician who treated the underprivileged in the smaller communities of Northern Ontario. Dr. Gretchen Roedde struggled with personal and humanitarian challenges. However, she accepted that the forces of nature always prevailed over life and death.

— *Dr. André Hurtubise, CCFP, FCFP*

Dr. Gretchen Roedde has worked in some of the world's toughest medical zones. In *Deep Water Dream* she brings her passion for medical justice to the Indigenous and working-class communities of Northern Ontario. Small town, country doctor memoir it ain't. This book is raw and real.

— *Charlie Angus, MP, Timmins–James Bay*

In this radical memoir of reconciliation — forty five years before *reconciliation* became a questionable buzzword — Gretchen Roedde writes of her education and life work as a doctor in the medically-underserved North. The "deep water" here flows out of the complex, lifelong relationships Gretchen has with her friends, mentors, patients, and colleagues in the Tema-Augama Anishnabai Nation. In a world of increasingly short thoughts and sharp polarities, here are the long thoughts of long lives, inspired by expansive dreams. The great power and healing here arise directly out of the lands, the waters, and the peoples of Northern Ontario.

— *Karen Connelly, therapist and author of* The Change Room

DEEP
WATER
DREAM

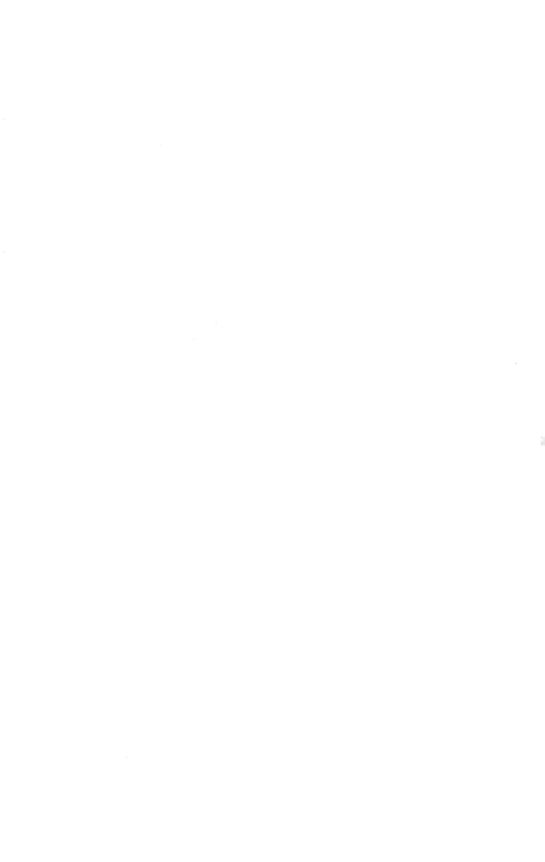

GRETCHEN ROEDDE

DEEP WATER DREAM

A MEDICAL VOYAGE
OF DISCOVERY IN
RURAL NORTHERN ONTARIO

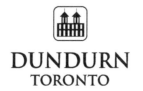

DUNDURN
TORONTO

Cover design: Laura Boyle
Printer: Webcom, a division of Marquis Book Printing Inc.

Library and Archives Canada Cataloguing in Publication

Roedde, Gretchen, author
    Deep water dream : a medical voyage of discovery in rural Northern
Ontario / Gretchen Roedde.

Issued in print and electronic formats.
ISBN 978-1-4597-4329-8 (softcover).--ISBN 978-1-4597-4330-4 (PDF).--
ISBN 978-1-4597-4331-1 (EPUB)

    1. Roedde, Gretchen. 2. Physicians--Ontario, Northern--Biography.
3. Medical care--Ontario, Northern. 4. Ontario, Northern--Rural conditions.
5. Autobiographies. I. Title.

FC3094.3.R66A3 2018   610.92   C2018-904994-4
                                                C2018-904995-2

1   2   3   4   5   22   21   20   19   18

 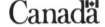 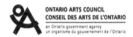

We acknowledge the support of the **Canada Council for the Arts**, which last year invested $153 million to bring the arts to Canadians throughout the country, and the **Ontario Arts Council** for our publishing program. We also acknowledge the financial support of the **Government of Ontario**, through the **Ontario Book Publishing Tax Credit** and the **Ontario Media Development Corporation**, and the **Government of Canada**.

Nous remercions le **Conseil des arts du Canada** de son soutien. L'an dernier, le Conseil a investi 153 millions de dollars pour mettre de l'art dans la vie des Canadiennes et des Canadiens de tout le pays.

Care has been taken to trace the ownership of copyright material used in this book. The author and the publisher welcome any information enabling them to rectify any references or credits in subsequent editions.

— *J. Kirk Howard, President*

The publisher is not responsible for websites or their content unless they are owned by the publisher.

Printed and bound in Canada.

VISIT US AT

 dundurn.com | 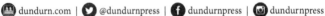 @dundurnpress | dundurnpress | dundurnpress

Dundurn
3 Church Street, Suite 500
Toronto, Ontario, Canada
M5E 1M2

For Jim, our children Anna and Alec,
and Hayley, Regan, and Etta

∽ Contents ∾

SECTION THREE

*SHA'NGABI'HANONG / shahn-guh-bee-han-noong /
Spirit Keeper of the West*

SECTION FOUR

*KEEWATINONG / key-weh-di-noong /
Spirit Keeper of the North*

∽ Foreword ∾

Having been asked to read Dr. Gretchen Roedde's book prior to publication and write something for her is an honour and a privilege. As I reflected on her first book, *A Doctor's Quest*, read this one, and pondered our relationship, what came to mind is a quote from Tom King, a well-known Indigenous author. "Stories are wonderful things and they are dangerous. Stories assert tremendous control over our lives, informing who we are and how we treat one another as friends, family and citizens. The truth about stories is that's all we are." I believe Gretchen's story is captured in this quote.

Not all who read this book will remember these stories the same way she does. Some will celebrate what they see of themselves and some may not. This is Gretchen's story to tell, and she does it well. She begins with her decision to go to medical school, describes the challenges of being a doctor, of her work with Treaty Nine, Bear Island, and in small Northern Ontario towns. She describes to us how her life as a doctor imposed on and affected her roles as a wife and a mother. As she weaves the story of her personal life with that of her professional life, we become very aware of her connection to people and her desire for a world where no one is left behind.

My friend has told her story and is sharing it with the world. It is a story of courage, to experience the unknown and to live life to its fullest even when you think you don't have the wherewithal to keep going.

As you read her book you will come to know the woman I know, a woman of great strength and ability. As I work to find words that describe her, I think of empathy, honour, humility, a force of nature, courage.

And I will close by saying *Meegwetch* to you, Gretchen, for your caring and service to humanity, for coming to my community, for being part of my life, but mostly for being my friend and for our times together.

— Victoria Grant, Loon Clan, Teme-Augama Anishnabai Qway (Deep Water Woman), and a member of the Temagami First Nation.
July 2018

∽ Introduction ℃

TEMAGAMI/TEMISKAMING IS THE ANISHINAABE WORD
TEMAGAMING: AT THE PLACE OF DEEP WATER.

This is a hopeful memoir, sharing my voyage of discovery as a mother, wife, and physician in several underserved (Indigenous, rural, Amish) communities in Northern Ontario; but it is also a difficult one, as these people have restricted access to health services that many Canadians take for granted. I am asking you to take this journey with me.

Indigenous Peoples in Canada have suicide rates twice as high as non-Indigenous people; in Inuit communities it's almost ten times higher.[1] One fifth of Canada's Indigenous Peoples live in Ontario. Indigenous youth in the province are more likely to be raised in single-parent families, to have higher rates of unemployment and poverty, and to be incarcerated than others in Ontario, often for trivial incidents taking parents away from their homes. This reflects deep-rooted racism in the justice system.[2] My non-Indigenous, poor patients in single-parent homes have these same high suicide and unemployment rates and substance abuse problems; it is poverty that is the determinant of health.

And there remains an underlying racism that we in Canada have to address more strongly. In the midst of my work decades ago in Sioux

Lookout Zone, tragedy divided the community — the racially moti-
vated murder of an Indigenous man. Understandably, our colleagues
were devastated. "It is a terrible thing. That poor man. He was peacefully sleeping off a night of drinking outside the Sioux hotel."

One Elder we were working with added, "He was killed by a bunch
of white kids, all sons of prominent families. They kicked him to death.
And then their parents have the nerve to try to get a Native rights lawyer
to work for them." The town was divided down racial lines. The white
refrain in town was that the boys shouldn't suffer for a foolish mistake
and lose their bright futures. Many First Nations concluded that this
was yet another racist murder.

Leaders in these communities are under tremendous pressures
and themselves have often had difficult childhoods with residential
schools, single parenting, and poverty. Alcohol was not unknown with
these chiefs. Gender-based violence occurred. I, myself, once experienced a colleague who was drunk and reached over and grabbed my
breast in a public gathering. I smiled through this challenge to the dignity of both of us and said nothing. I was to start medical school the
next year. This work was important to me; it was why I was going to
train to be a doctor. Again, this is not culturally specific. In 75 percent
of the developing countries I work in, the majority of women think
gender-based violence is acceptable.

Many of the efforts to provide health care to Indigenous Peoples
have been colonial and destructive of culture, and yet it is the strengths
of community and tradition that have proved the most promising in
helping to build First Nations, Inuit, and Métis identities and close the
gaps in health status with non-Indigenous people in Canada.[3] When
well-meaning non-Indigenous governments sent in teams of crisis
workers to an isolated community in the midst of an epidemic of suicide attempts, insufficient consultation with the chiefs and councils
took place. These workers did not have long-term experience in non-
Indigenous communities. It was the time of the spring goose hunt. The
whole community — everyone, all ages, even the dogs — set out at night
for the annual traditional celebration. In the morning, the surprised

crisis workers wondered where everyone had gone. Out on the goose hunt, in the midst of a community's grief, there were chuckles about how the health workers were faring alone in the community.

As a non-Indigenous person writing with my own voice and through my own lens and observed experiences with other cultures, I have made many mistakes. Different worlds have subtleties in senses of humour and nuances of words that cannot be translated, which can create errors of substance and tone. I have tried to correct these with input from the original speakers, but any remaining mistakes or misinterpretations are my own. Similarly, French-Canadian and Amish communities use the English language differently.

In underserved ethnic minorities, it is the members of the communities themselves that create the strongest parts of the health care team. Whether white or First Nations, neighbourhood people, in my experience, make the lives of dying people, birthing women, or ill people at all stages of their lives more meaningful and more bearable. Whether helping a Cree community develop a medical vocabulary in their own language, training Indigenous people as community-based health workers, or bringing a priest to a house call to minister to a dying French-Canadian woman, I have learned that the boundaries between physician and community are redrawn to strengthen families and their ability to care for their loved ones. Because culture itself is a determinant of health,[4] respecting culture and spirituality and building on them will improve health outcomes,[5] for example, working with midwives caring for the Amish minority community as they deliver their children in a home-like setting close to hospital.

The issues of faith in the midst of adversity, whether professional or personal, are powerful themes in this reflective and complex memoir of joyful resilience. People who live their commitment to social justice are celebrated, whether they fight for land claims or to bring quality palliative care to all Canadians. It was a member of Parliament serving Timmins–James Bay, where much of the book is situated, who was able to bring consensus in the House of Commons.

"Today in the House of Commons, we have all main parties, especially the government, standing up on the need to establish a pan-Canadian palliative care strategy," Charlie Angus told journalists after the May 28, 2014, vote. "This is very important. It says that this government and the federal Parliament of Canada recognize the importance of palliative care and helping find better strategies.…"

Canadian Conference of Catholic Bishops president Archbishop Paul-André Durocher [formerly the parish priest in my home town] said he rejoiced at "such a clear signal that gathers voices from all across the country in recognizing the need for good, quality care to help people, those who are dying and those who care for them in a way that is consistent with a life ethic."

"I congratulate Mr. Charlie Angus in bringing this forward," the archbishop said. "I hope that the Canadian government will take this sign seriously and will seek to move this project forward in any way possible."[6]

Structured in four sections with the four compass points, colours, and themes of the Medicine Wheel in Anishinaabe culture, this book explores the challenges and joys of a doctor committed to social justice working with marginalized communities in Northern Ontario. The title, *Deep Water Dream*, reflects life in Indigenous communities (such as on Lake Temagami) as well as rural general practice on Lake Temiskaming, providing home-based palliative care, midwifery support to the Amish, and family medicine to underserved groups in a harsh climate with major weather and transport challenges between levels of care. Both Temagami and Temiskaming mean At the Place of Deep Water in Anishinaabe. Each chapter reflects themes from the Medicine Wheel — animal totems, plants, and spiritual challenges — so, for example, Section 1, *Wabanong,* or Spirit Keeper of the East, is represented by the colour yellow and the season of spring and new beginnings. The totem animal is eagle, which flies high, seeking illumination regarding your life path and giving inspiration to begin. The chapters "Baptism," "East Is the Time of Spring and New Beginnings," "True Home in the Spirit," and "Eagle Overhead" reflect these themes.

Section 2, *Shawanong*, or Spirit Keeper of the South, continues with chapters reflecting on my work with Indigenous people while raising a family: "Blueberry Girl," "Learning to Trust," and "Windigo Welcome," among others; Section 3, *Sha'ngabi'hanong*, or Spirit Keeper of the West, segues into my medical life in non-Indigenous communities, including palliative care and in delivering the Amish with the midwives: "*Makwa* (Bear) Goes Within," "Grace-Filled Fall," "Cedar Grounding," and "A Jubilant Birth." And finally, Section 4, *Keewatinong*, or Spirit Keeper of the North, reflects a time of rebirth and of understanding, giving thanks for our blessings, and sharing the gifts of experience. The cycle of family and community renews in the final four chapters, "Moose on the Red Squirrel Road," "Gift Giving," "Sweetgrass," and "Winter Wisdom."

I should point out that the names of patients and colleagues in *Deep Water Dream* are a mix of actual and altered names. All patients have given consent for their stories to be shared. On occasion, events that occurred over several seasons have been compressed into one for the purposes of flow and focus.

NOTES

1. Saman Khan, "Aboriginal Mental Health: The Statistical Reality," *Visions Journal* 5, no. 1 (2008), heretohelp.bc.ca/visions/aboriginal-people-vol5/aboriginal-mental-health-the-statistical-reality.
2. Noelle Spotton, "A Profile of Aboriginal Peoples in Ontario," (background paper, Ipperwash Inquiry, n.d.) p. 3, attorneygeneral.jus.gov.on.ca/inquiries/ipperwash/policy_part/research/pdf/Spotton_Profile-of-Aboriginal-Peoples-in-Ontario.pdf.
3. Peter L. Twohig, review of *Aboriginal Health in Canada*, by James B. Waldram, D. Ann Herring, and T. Kue Young, *Acadiensis* 32, no. 1 (Autumn 2002), journals.lib.unb.ca/index.php/acadiensis/article/view/10714/11425.

4. Melissa Sweet, "Culture Is an Important Determinant of Health: Professor Ngiare Brown at NACCHO Summit," *Crikey* (blog), August 20, 2013, blogs.crikey.com.au/croakey/2013/08/20/culture-is-an-important-determinant-of-health-professor-ngiare-brown-at-naccho-summit.

5. Prof. Ngi Brown, "Exploring Determinants of Health and Wellbeing," (slide presentation, Lowitja Institute Roundtable, November 2014), lowitja.org.au/sites/default/files/docs/Ngaire-Brown.pdf.

6. Charlie Angus, quoted in Deborah Gyapong, "House of Commons Adopts Angus Motion on Palliative Care," *Catholic Register*, May 28, 2014, catholicregister.org/item/18262-house-of-commons-adopts-angus-motion-on-palliative-care.

SECTION ONE

WABANONG / wah-buh-noong /
Spirit Keeper of the East

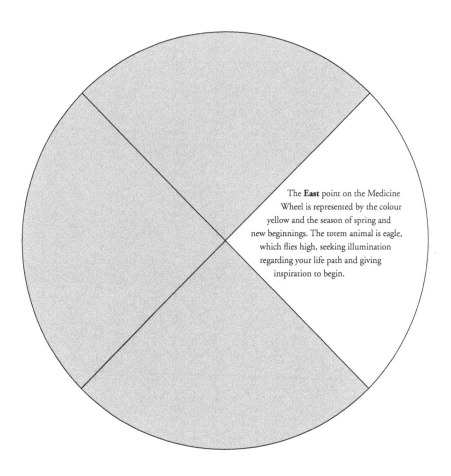

The **East** point on the Medicine Wheel is represented by the colour yellow and the season of spring and new beginnings. The totem animal is eagle, which flies high, seeking illumination regarding your life path and giving inspiration to begin.

1

BAPTISM, 1973

BAPTISM, GIVEN: *SEGAHUNDAH-GAWIN*

BAPTISM, RECEIVED: *SEGAHUN-DAHGOOWIN*

BAPTIZE: *SEGAHUNDAHGA*

BAPTIZED, HE IS B.: *SEGAHUN-DAHSO*

"Abinoojii." "To be lifted up" is a better explanation than "child," which is another translation. An Anishinaabe phrase from Wikwemikong, a community that is home to three languages, Bea Shawanda spoke it firmly. She was directing me, as a child, to find my own inner strength for what was ahead. This simple but powerful expression said to her lovingly by the family, Sophie and Eli, who raised her was now said by Bea to me, "Child. You will be lifted up." She was trying to prepare me to go up north.

But Bea still had questions.

"Why do you think we should let you help us? What gifts are you bringing to us? I am the bridge between the people and you coming to us to help. I need to explain you to the Chiefs. If we bring in non-Native resources, like you in health and social services, we have to help you bridge." She spoke angrily.

I felt threatened. I had never been up north, in isolated First Nations communities. I knew nothing about these communities. I had met Bea when I was volunteering with her group in Toronto, working with homeless Indigenous people. She had asked me to help with Grand Council Treaty No. 9, a new Indigenous organization representing the northern half of the province of Ontario, in Canada. Its goal was to set up a First Nations paramedic training program for a group of OjiCree communities in the Windigo Tribal Council, north of Sioux Lookout, in northwestern Ontario, and to set up alternatives to jail for addicted youth. She had invited me to this Chiefs' Conference in Thunder Bay to start meeting the people I would be working with. It was true. What gifts did I bring?

We were in our hotel room. I was rocking one of Bea's kids, Maheengun, in my arms, swaying rhythmically and pretending not to feel worried about my inexperience. I kept my face neutral and left the hotel room, still rocking Maheengun. Pint-size dynamo (maybe five feet?) Bea still argued forcefully beside me, asking me about my commitment as we took the elevator to the large conference room on the ground floor.

I looked across the room and shook my head, tossing my dark blond hair loosely over my shoulders. There was one other non-Indigenous person there, a good-looking, dark-haired guy with a moustache. I couldn't help but notice him. He wore a green plaid Viyella shirt with brown corduroy pants and closed-toe wooden clogs. He nodded at me, unsmiling, from the other side of the large, smoke-filled room, as a confusion of voices — Cree, OjiCree, English — hummed through the haze. He seemed totally unfazed by the chaos. I had no idea I was staring at my future husband.

———

I had started off as a physical anthropology student at the University of Toronto planning to study primates in Gibraltar in the summer. Instead, I switched to social anthropology and had sessions that looked at various ethnic minority cultures around the world. One day, a guest lecturer, a Cree leader, spoke of the symptoms of the pain of his people,

violent and accidental deaths, drinking, and drugs, babies born with
fetal alcohol syndrome. I went up to him after the lecture. "Is there
anything I can do to help?" He looked down at me, grinning broadly.
"We actually don't need your kind of help. But if you're serious, call Bea
Shawanda. She lives in Toronto. She is the new head of the Treaty No. 9
health program. But I am pretty sure we don't need more anthropolo-
gists. Ever thought of becoming a doctor? That would be more helpful
to us. Till we train more of our own."

I left, making room for the throng of mostly female students
crowding around him, being charmed by his smiles and tanned coppery-
skinned good looks.

I took his advice. I did look up Bea Shawanda and worked with
her for several months. I met her kids, Byron, Elizabeth, and the baby
Maheengun. Bea invited me to prepare to go farther north. And I
applied to medical school. So I was there, in Thunder Bay, at the Treaty
No. 9 Chiefs' Conference, at her invitation from a few weeks earlier. At
the conference for the Chiefs the sessions moved slowly, with translation
back and forth between Cree, OjiCree, and English. About ten of the
one hundred people in the smoky room were women. The men were
all clean-shaven, except for that white guy with the moustache. A few
wore beaded deerskin jackets. I was trying to take in every detail. I kept
Maheengun in my arms, as Bea was busy building relationships and
camaraderie, laughing with the Chiefs, engaging them with her ideas
for social programs, drug and alcohol worker training, and a paramedic
program. *Abinoojii.* Did I have the skills to rise to this challenge?

I survived that first difficult week. Back in Toronto, Bea and I met
at her home. Bea explained: you need to be confident that you have
skills to share with us. You need to know that people may be angry
with you as a non-Native person helping us. "I needed to see how you
would react. What you'd do if people in the communities say challeng-
ing things to you. You will not be working for the white world. You will
not be staying with the teachers or at the nursing station. You'll be living
and travelling with our people. Our people have a lot of anger with the
white world. I, myself, had bad experiences in the residential schools. I

went to school when I was four and a half. These schools were used as orphanages. It was there I first experienced violence. My mom had died when I was two, and I was adopted within my family. I worked through those difficult years by becoming an activist. That was part of the healing process for me."

Bea looked up at me, a novel experience as I am only 5 feet 4 inches tall myself. She had had tuberculosis in her spine as a kid. She spent months in the TB sanatorium. She remembers feeling frightened of the janitors. She couldn't walk for a while and was told she could never have kids. She proved the doctors wrong and had borne the children she was raising. She sure was raising me in a new world, too.

"I think you'll be okay because you are working for us. I was taught that in the first five years, a child receives what they need, including courage of heart. *Abinoojii.* I hope it is the same in your culture. You should have the strength you will need."

I "passed." Bea and the chiefs had agreed I could travel and work as a volunteer for Treaty No. 9. My travel expenses were paid and were extensive as most of the communities are fly-in.

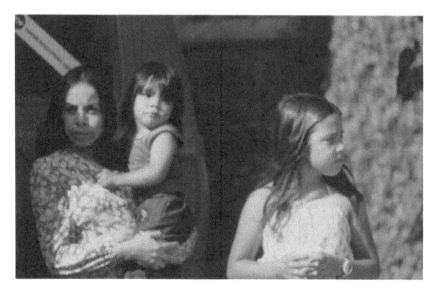

Bea Shawanda with her son, Maheengun, and daughter, Elizabeth, 1974.

In the summer of 1974, I lived with Bea, her sons, and her daughter, Elizabeth, in Timmins. I had finished my B.A. in anthropology; in the fall I was going to medical school. Bea already felt like family. After working in the head office in Timmins to prepare, this feisty woman and I travelled with her kids to spend a week at Bea's home community, Wikwemikong. She was Odawa, one of the three Nations that comprise the Wikwemikong community (with Ojibwe and Pottawotomie) on Manitoulin Island (Mnidoo Mnis).

Wikwemikong is the largest community — the "fourth stopping place" — on Mnidoo Mnis. According to history recorded both orally and on birchbark scrolls, the Anishinaabe people had been led by spiritual clan leaders, *miigis,* to migrate west along the St. Lawrence. The first stopping place was small Turtle Island, now Montreal, followed by Niagara Falls, then Detroit, and then Manitoulin. The entire North American continent is seen as a large Turtle Island in Anishinaabe mythology.

Bea was related to most of the people we met. *"Ahnii!"* shouted various relatives, greeting us in Odawa. Her kids were cheerfully meeting cousins, and outfits were finalized for dancing at the powwow, full skirts overlaid with small bells, elaborately braided hair, deerskin shirts and leggings. I struggled to learn a few simple steps of a round dance and joined in the powwow. Wikwemikong is large, with three thousand people on reserve and more who live off reserve. In between dance practices and meals of fried baloney, corn on the cob, and fry bread, we visited the local seniors' home, where everyone, staff and residents alike, was First Nations. In the health centre, a mix of Western and traditional medicine was in use. We met with health workers and community members at the general medical clinic who were upset about the recent spate of teenage suicide attempts, many of which had been "completed."

After training in the United States, Bea had become the first Indigenous leader to in eastern Canada to set up drug and alcohol programs. She wanted to expand both treatment and prevention options. Bea left her kids with her Treaty 9 family in Timmins. We were freer now to travel and drove south from Timmins for several hours, looking at alternatives to incarceration for Treaty 9 area youth with drug and alcohol offences. We stopped in for a couple of hours at Project Dare, which was modelled on Outward Bound. The goal of this centre was to give troubled young teens a chance to learn about themselves as individuals and to rely on their team to exceed their limits. A centre like this could help to prevent substance abuse.

We drove onto the grounds late one afternoon in early summer. A mixed stand of maples and pines swayed gently in a light breeze above our heads. We scrambled down a winding path to look across at a rocky slope farther along the escarpment. Six young people were learning to rappel against the cliff, swinging on complicated ropes and harnesses. Their feet scrambled for footholds as they descended. Two others were trying to climb up the rocks, laughing with each other. At the base of the cliff on the shore, another group of three were getting a canoe ready for a voyage.

The director came out of a one-storey building to meet us. After we introduced ourselves, he explained the theory of the program. "These kids have had a lot of tough experiences, and the adults around them were often not trustworthy because of drinking and other problems. So it's a huge transformation for these young adults to learn how to rely on each other."

Bea explained what Treaty 9 was doing. "I'm the director of Health and Social Programs. We are training workers for the National Native Alcohol and Drug Abuse Program. That is one step for First Nations people to have someone of our own culture to help stop addiction. But the cycle is hard to break. Young people whose parents are drinking learn this early as a coping strategy. We're trying to find safe places where our young people can learn to be self-confident, to live in the bush, and to help each other in positive ways."

I could not imagine communities where no one had running water, all lived in poor housing, and alcohol abuse and gas sniffing were common. How could this be happening in the wealthy province of Ontario, in the rich country of Canada? In 1974, the reality facing First Nations had been largely neglected in the media. I was glad to be travelling with

Bea and her kids, who were cheerful and optimistic as I became pain-fully aware of truths they had always known.

After another hour of touring the facility and asking how Treaty 9 youth could access services like Project Dare, we drove to our next stop, Cecil Facer, a minimum-security institution for youth. It was an early evening in late June when we arrived at the main buildings. I was a bit scared. Although minimum-security, this was still basically a prison. How angry might these kids be toward white people like me?

The sun was just setting as we arrived. The sky was turning a deep blue violet. The dark red sun slipped below the horizon. The officer in charge smiled uncertainly and led us into a large informal room. About twelve people were there, a mix of staff and inmates who had just fin-ished their supper. The youth workers were a bit hip, casually dressed. The Indigenous kids seemed shy and avoided eye contact. The white kids were equally hesitant to speak.

Bea took the lead, explaining why we were here. "We have a lot of kids raised by families who had little parenting skills. Their parents suffered through the residential schools, where they were beaten if they spoke their own language. They were cut off from their own traditions. Some of them spent years in TB hospitals. It is not surprising that they had a hard time being good parents. So their kids get drunk, take drugs, and break the law. Now some end up in jail south of Timmins. We want to try to set up a place where they won't get into trouble, where both they and their communities are safe. Where they can still go to school. An alternative to jail."

Two of the white kids started to laugh quietly, off to one side. They were both heavily tattooed.

"This is no jail. It's easy to break out of here. We skip out for the night or a few days. These 'guards' are no match for us."

"Hey, settle down you guys! Don't tell these strangers all your secrets!" joked one of the youth workers, who was dressed in jeans, his name badge on a string around his neck. Bea and I took careful notes: what it would take to create a combination educational boarding facil-ity, with traditional skills building (trapping, canoeing) to help troubled

Indigenous teens. We weren't worried about kids getting away. We just wanted them to have a place to go that wasn't prison, somewhere safe for them to sort themselves out.

———

Thirty years later, in 2003, I was working as a general practitioner (GP) in the Northern Ontario community of Kirkland Lake. I had fulfilled my earlier goal: I had gone north to become a GP. I did locums in small towns, and I had worked in more remote communities in the far north with Indigenous Peoples and in poor countries overseas. This was a one-week assignment in Kirkland Lake, a mining town down on its luck, with at least one bar at every intersection and the occasional drunken fight on those same corners.

In the clinic where I was working, drug addicts would come in with a variety of tales to explain why they needed their narcotic prescription filled earlier than it was due. I had heard that the GP I was replacing had had his car trashed by local drug dealers because he had started to cut off the prescriptions for people who did not need OxyContin, Percocet, or morphine. He had succumbed to the scare tactics and begun reordering narcotics without asking questions.

In the midst of a busy day in the office, with five minutes allotted per patient and a waiting room overfilled with people, the next person brought into the examining room was a dark-haired, angular, brown-faced young man. His feet were shackled together. He did not meet my eyes. In my white world we expect eye contact. In Indigenous communities, eyes are often averted out of shyness, politeness, or respect. He wore a pastel-coloured jumpsuit. This sixteen-year-old Cree youth, from up the west coast of James Bay, was handcuffed to a police guard.

"Go on, Stan. Tell the doc what's wrong with you!" exclaimed the cop.

Stan said nothing, just looked down, so the cop replied on his behalf. "He keeps coughing. He was checked for TB before we brought him into custody. It's been over a week now. Maybe check him out for pneumonia?"

I listened to his breathing; there were reduced breath sounds in his lower left lung. I thought he did have pneumonia and gave him a prescription for antibiotics and a requisition for a chest X-ray.

———

There were still no good options for Indigenous kids who had drug and alcohol charges. The incarceration rate for Indigenous Peoples is ten times higher than for other Canadians. They make up less than 5 percent of the total population in the country but nearly one quarter of the jailed population. More than 20 percent of all federally incarcerated Indigenous offenders are twenty-five years of age or younger, as compared to just over 12 percent of non-Indigenous offenders. So these kids from up the coast of James Bay, the ones we had been trying to help in 1973–74, were still troubled and being jailed for minor offences.

Fort Albany, Attawapiskat, Fort Severn, Moose Factory — these are wild and free places, home to geese flying overhead and the northern lights cascading through the skies. But Stan had no freedom. This young man was beginning his adult life in prison. These young people had been charged with minor drug and alcohol offences yet began their adult lives as prisoners in poorly-equipped, white-dominated prisons. It didn't matter that the white people called the places "institutions." It didn't matter that most of the white people in my waiting room were requesting narcotics yet had managed to avoid drug and alcohol charges. It didn't matter that many Indigenous youth used substances to bury the pain of their earlier memories of sexual or physical abuse.

———

But in 1974, my dream was how all this was going to be changed.

We made our way to the room we were sharing in Cecil Facer's residence. We jotted a few quick notes and talked quietly as we packed to go back to Timmins the next morning. "I think we'll be able to do this. We'll need funding. We'll need to do a lot of work. But this should be a priority for help from government," explained Bea. It was several hours of driving back to Timmins, and then the following week, in 1974, Bea, her eleven-year-old daughter, Elizabeth, and I took our first trip to Sioux Lookout.

I loved standing on the steps of the aircraft with Elizabeth at my side; she and I leaned into each other, smiling shyly; she was like my little sister. Bea was both sister and mother. Elizabeth and I wore blue jeans, long-sleeved T-shirts, and delicately beaded necklaces. Mine was white and lilac. Ever one to adopt external cultural trappings, I topped it off with a rain jacket with an embroidered First Nations design.

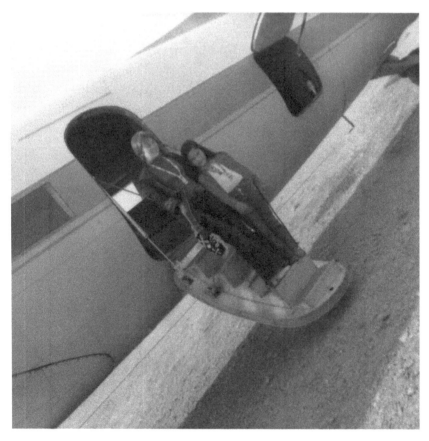

Gretchen Roedde and Elizabeth Edgar, Sioux Lookout Zone, 1974.

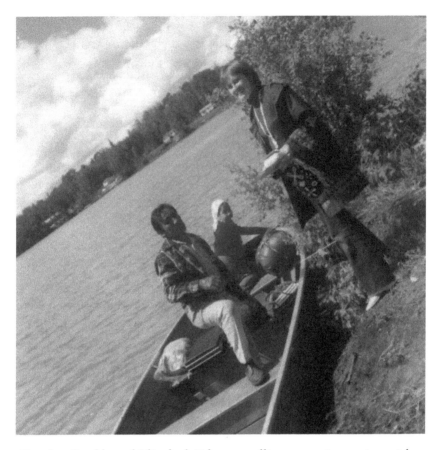

*Gretchen Roedde and Elizabeth Edgar travelling to nursing station with
an OjiCree leader, Sandy Lake, 1974.*

After two days of meetings in Sioux Lookout with the hospital doctors, we flew on Bearskin Airlines to Sandy Lake in a blue-and-white
six-seater Cessna 180 floatplane. Then, a plaid-jacketed OjiCree leader
took us by open steel boat to visit the nursing station, a pale green
one-storey prefab building. Elizabeth and I stood together, the lake glistening behind us, the rocks and grasses beneath our feet, before going in
to greet the hard-working nurses.

I was in a cross-cultural middle and muddle. I did feel "not white."
I had no kinship with the white nurses who had flush toilets while the

First Nations people used outhouses and drank lake water polluted by the raw sewage from the teacherage and nursing station. But I had no experience with the OjiCree culture or language. In communities where the professional teachers and nurses were white, I had made my choice. I was working for the people, or *Anishinaabeg*, the Anishinaabe word for people. I stayed with them in simple one-room log buildings and hauled water. Bea had introduced me to Frank Beardy, a cheerful bear of a man working for Treaty 9 with whom I was to travel. I met another white woman who had also taken sides. Paulette Giles played guitar and sang at a lively evening night out in Sandy Lake. Later she was to become a successful writer. She was helping the communities to set up radio, television, and print media services on their own terms, what would become Wawatay News.

The next day we boarded another Bearskin flight, this time to Big Trout Lake. I stayed with Frank's sister, Virginia. As we got ready for bed, someone started to bang on the door and shout in OjiCree with a slurred voice. Virginia laughed. "Just a guy who had too much to drink. The door is locked. He won't bother us. He's just shouting 'Let me in! I want a woman! Open the door!' But he'll go away when we turn the lights out. Don't worry." I was glad I was staying with Virginia. I would have been scared if this had happened and I was staying with other white women, and no one knew the language.

I tried to relax as I fell asleep.

Two days later we flew to Deer Lake. We had a loose schedule to travel to many of these satellite communities. Weather in these smaller settlements could keep us stuck for a week or more. In another small community, Kasabonika, we spent one such week, and it was here that I discovered I was described in OjiCree as a *mashkikiiwikwe*. This word suggests someone with medical or nursing training who is a white person and a woman. I was not that person. I had an anthropology degree and as a student had evaluated a First Nations paramedic training program in northern Manitoba the previous summer. Though I was about to start medical school, I was no *mashkikiiwikwe*.

When a panicked First Nations community health worker named Evelyn came to find me because a man was unable to pee after two days, I had no idea what to do. We had tried to raise the nurse in Sioux Lookout Zone on the radio phone and got nothing but squawk and squelch. I read the labels on his medicine bottles. I reasoned that Hydrodiuril was probably a diuretic. I tried that. He managed to pee after three hours, and I now had first hand experience of what these Community Health Representatives had to cope with — many with barely grade seven education or less, no clinical training, and days without skilled backup. Years later, this experience would serve me in good stead when I was revising training programs to better equip these workers for the challenges of their isolated settings. While I was in medical school for the next few years, I would send clothes up to Evelyn. She wanted them for the community, and my fellow medical students kept me supplied. In exchange, Evelyn sent me a lovely beaded deerskin bag, which I still have, though it is now proudly displayed in my clinic up north.

Being weathered-in meant coming to understand something of nature's rhythms. This was not something I had much experience with. I prided myself on my organizational skills. I had planned how many communities I would visit over several weeks, writing down the details in a small notebook — where we would go, how long we would stay, who we would interview in each community, and a rough list of interview questions. Bea and Elizabeth had been joined by two other leaders: Frank Beardy, from northwestern Ontario, and George Maclean, a Cree from up the James Bay coast whose fair colouring reflected his Scottish Hudson's Bay Company roots. When he saw my careful notes, Frank started laughing. "You can't plan like that! The weather will decide. You might get stuck somewhere you didn't expect, and you'll learn what you can there. Then there might be some fishermen who can give you a lift on a plane to somewhere you didn't think you were going to visit. You have to stay a lot looser than you are now!" It was invaluable advice for life in the North — in fact, an important way to look at life anywhere.

Our small group flew into one reserve that Frank had not visited for many years. Yet it was a place he knew well; it was an offshoot of the village in which he had grown up. The newly created community had needed a store, and as a twelve-year-old boy he'd been sent to run it. He stayed there, away from his family, for many months, sorting out supplies, making orders, and selling basic foodstuffs and materials. Because people remembered him, I expected excited rejoicings and catching up. But the adults passed quietly, greeting him with small smiles. "*Ahnee*," they said, shyly, discreetly.

I learned to haul water, a job I shared with a young man with Down syndrome, who earned a few cents doing this task for others — an honoured role. As a woman, I was expected to cook for everyone. Bea showed me how to use the propane burner to make a perennial favourite: chicken bought frozen from the Hudson's Bay store for an astronomical price and fried in bacon grease. She delegated this task to me before she flew back to Timmins, having decided I would be okay without her. Woman to woman, non-white to white. I felt honoured.

Right after getting stuck in Kasabonika, we got weathered-in, in Wunnumin Lake, for a few days. In Wunnumin Lake, I met Frank's family. His sisters taught me to play cards late into the night. After several weeks, I was accustomed to their love of teasing. Frank Beardy had taught me the phrase *onizhishin gidiy* in order for me to greet the Chiefs properly. I practised a few times with Frank. As I carefully pronounced the words, I became suspicious of his quivering lower lip and the crinkling laugh lines at the corners of his eyes. I quietly took his sister Virginia aside. Frank had told me this meant "Pleased to meet you," and he'd explained it would be courteous to greet the Chief in this way. Luckily, I had learned to double-check facts such as these, and when I asked Virginia what this phrase meant, she laughed out loud. Turns out, I narrowly avoided telling the Chief he had a nice ass. My near miss still made people laugh, because everyone was expecting me to say *onizhishin gidiy*. The moccasin telegraph, I learned, was extremely effective. In community after community, women Elders wearing flowered kerchiefs would come up to me chuckling, teasing me with *onizhishin gidiy*.

To return to the head office of Treaty No. 9, in Timmins, Bea and Elizabeth and I flew Bearskin Airlines, first to Sioux Lookout, then to Thunder Bay, and then on to Timmins in the northeast. Here, I officially met the historian working on hunting and fishing rights and treaty research, Jim, whom I had seen across the crowded Chiefs' Conference room in Thunder Bay a few months earlier. Still with a dark brown moustache and longish brown hair, he rushed out of the office with a cheery wave. "Come for supper sometime?"

Sure, I thought. Bea had already told me that Treaty 9 leaders frowned on interracial dating in the office. In fact, staff of any culture could not have relationships with clients — that is, with the Chiefs and communities — as part of the Treaty 9 work ethic. Jim was handsome, smart, and white. The day after we met, I spent a weekend with friends farther south, in Kenabeek (*ginebic* is snake in Anishinaabe), near Haileybury and New Liskeard. I drove down with another summer student, Cathy Beamish, who was training to be a lawyer. "You'll like my friends, Gretchen! Christine and Henry live in the bush with their kids. She has a huge garden, and Henry plays banjo."

I came back to Timmins with an armload of salad greens from their garden to bring to that first dinner with Jim. A great cook, he'd prepared "Captain's Chicken," with mild curry spices and homemade bread to accompany my salad. He asked after my friends in Kenabeek.

"I'll look them up sometime. I'm doing work for the Bear Island Band land claim down on Lake Temagami, even though it's not part of Treaty 9. That's just a bit south of Kenabeek. You say Henry plays banjo? That's great. I play bluegrass guitar and Dobro with friends like Chief Gary Potts from Temagami First Nation. Maybe we can get together sometime and play with your friend Henry."

A few nights after we met, I dreamt we were walking up a long staircase, and the Pope was at the top, marrying us. After that summer, I started medical school at McMaster University, in Hamilton.

If Bea had brought me into her world, other teachers blessed me on my way forward as a doctor. At my medical school interview, the interview team (a medical student, professor, community physician, and a woman who represented the "public") asked me about my goals.

"I'm from Thunder Bay, and I want to go north to work with Indigenous Peoples."

The panel laughed. Apparently, the *Globe and Mail* had just run a story on this new medical school, McMaster, in which the editorial read that the typical Mac student is twenty-three, female, from Thunder Bay, with a B.A., not a science background, and wants to work with Indigenous people. I had a pretty tough grilling, but that really was who I was, and I got in.

Once there, though, I was unsure of myself. My new teachers were mostly "staff men"; they wore white coats and stern frowns with their stethoscopes. Although McMaster had a reputation for innovative learning, many of our professors were old school and enjoyed ridiculing the students. We would cringe at Grand Rounds, hoping not to be noticed and asked by our instructors to stand up in front of a huge auditorium full of doctors at various stages of practice and training, to hesitantly explain exactly what was going on in a chest X-ray or cardiogram. Although half of us were women, these more traditional physicians weren't sure what to make of us.

We women were slightly afraid and regularly intimidated by these staff men. One day, I had to explain to a young family that their ten-year-old son had a serious form of leukemia, and the aggressive treatments he would receive might not save his life. Later, the presiding physician gave me feedback on my performance: "Your lower lip trembled when you gave them the news. You have to be more professional! You're just too sentimental."

Another of our staff men was a crusty cardiologist. He would parade along the wards followed by a clutch of eager, nervous white-jacketed medical students. He seemed to enjoy barking out commands. "I want arterial blood gases on this man. Every day!"

The patient was an Irish Catholic father of two young daughters. He lay dying in his hospital bed, clutching a holy medal and a rosary. "Please, I just want to go home. I know I'm dying. I want to spend my last days with my wife and children!"

The cardiologist refused. "We have to do more tests. You have a viral infection in your heart; it's failing. But you're too young to talk about dying. You're only in your fifties."

So every day we had to take blood for the blood gases, at times stabbing his groin or neck when it got too hard to take the sample from the artery in his wrist and still taking blood from a vein in his arm to check other aspects of his health. But we no longer did ward rounds on him, that time-honoured ritual of the senior doctor parading around the ward expounding wisdom. "Nothing we can do for him anyway," grunted this cardiologist.

I could barely contain my anger. Through clenched teeth, I asked "Why, then, do we keep taking blood on him?"

"I want to see how his kidneys are holding up. We have to keep checking his potassium levels and his digoxin levels, as well as how much oxygen he has in his blood," the doctor replied in measured tones.

I wanted to shout "He just wants to go home to die!" but I kept silent, because the reproving look was answer enough. I thought back to my first degree, in anthropology, when I had done an elective on medical ethics, which included the rights of the dying to know they are dying, and to an essay I did on Cicely Saunders, who founded the palliative care movement in England. We were so far behind in Canada. When this poor man died the following week, our resident was asked to go in to convince the weeping widow to let us do an autopsy, so we could see how damaged the heart was. She refused our wish as we had refused theirs.

If dying was a medical business, so, too, was being born. The first time I went into the Obstetrics (OB) ward to observe a birth, I had to go through an elaborate routine of scrubbing my hands and arms for ten minutes. Then I was gowned up in several layers of greens, gloved, masked, and given sterile green booties to put over my shoes. At one point, my elbow touched the gown of an OB nurse who wore greens but was not "sterile." The command came immediately from the senior obstetrician, who did not even glance at me as he barked, "Out, re-scrub, re-gown, and glove." Another student quickly stepped into my spot, delighting in my absence as he now had the better view.

In every hospital delivery I observed during that time (1974–77), the mother was given an epidural and required at least "outlet forceps" to deliver. When a woman has had an epidural, she can no longer feel the pain of labour, but she also has no sensation telling her to push. Forceps are two interlocking metal blades that are inserted into the vaginal "outlet" and held by the doctor to grasp the baby's head and pull the baby out. One intervention, like an epidural, usually leads to another intervention, such as forceps or surgery, to deliver the baby. If the head is too high because labour has stalled out early, it is not possible to use forceps as the head cannot be reached, and if the labour is not progressing, an operative delivery, or Caesarean section, is needed. Medicine seemed too much in control. Was there no other way to arrive and to leave this earth?

The one-hundred-hour workweeks were starting to wear me down. Jim and I lived together the year before we married with the support of my parish priest, who suggested we had a tough life ahead with our commitment to our careers and the distance apart. Jim was working in Timmins while I was at medical school in Hamilton. We needed to check out whether this would actually work before we got married.

We had a great support system as Jim's outstanding parents lived in nearby Ancaster. His dad, James, was a science professor at McMaster, and his mom, Irene, was a retired social worker known for her ability to feed forty at a moment's notice:

"Irene, we have several post-docs, visiting professors, and students in town. I'm bringing them for supper; we'll be there about six p.m. No Muslims, so cook whatever you like, and alcohol is definitely permissible!"

Jim and I were frequent visitors to his parents' home and enjoyed great family meals with his extended family of four other siblings and their spouses. They all provided us with great friendships throughout the challenges of medical training and our later work up north.

Jim was commuting back and forth from the Treaty 9 office in Timmins to Hamilton, where we lived. Once, on a rare weekend off, we had travelled north of Quebec to a conference on Indigenous history with his colleague Harry Achneepineskum, from Attawapiskat. Harry's mom was a powerful Medicine Woman. She could tell families where the drowned bodies of their loved ones could be found. Harry's dad made Jim and me pairs of long, curved snowshoes. Forty years later, my pair still carries me over the drifted snow.

Driving into Quebec City, Harry quietly announced, "I had a dream last month before coming on this trip. I will die soon, by fire."

As we drove, listening to Harry, Jim and I looked at each other. We did not speak. Jim was driving and kept his eyes on the road. Back then, we could still speak with silent glances. I looked at Harry and told him that we were honoured he had told us this story. "If this is how your journey will end, we'll keep your memory close in our hearts. We will be in sorrow but will be grateful for our time together and the fact that you have been told in advance. If this is how your Medicine Wheel is turning, the dream helps us all to be prepared."

Over the next few months, Jim and I kept up with our busy schedules. After deciding that we could manage our complex lives, we were married one year later, in the summer of 1975, when Jim was twenty-eight and I was twenty-three. There was great rejoicing in a Roman Catholic celebration at the University of Toronto attended by family, friends, medical students, and Indigenous colleagues. Cathy Beamish was our maid of honour. Bea and her kids were there; her youngest son, Maheengun, danced next to the priest at the front of the church. We had a potluck feast, Bach on the piano, and a bluegrass band playing "Haste to the Wedding." The priest took a turn at the fiddle, and the square dancing went on long into the night. Chief Gary Potts from Bear Island sent us a deep purple Hudson's Bay blanket as a wedding gift.

Over the next few months, Jim was in touch with Harry. We learned that he had started to prepare to leave the earth. He finished some work at the university where he was studying, sorting through his possessions as he did so.

One of Harry's projects was fighting a proposed hydroelectric power dam. This involved flying into remote communities to get their views and to share their concerns regarding migrating animals and fish should the great rivers be dammed. During one trip, the plane Harry was flying in hit heavy weather. Huge storms engulfed the plane; visibility dropped. The pilot descended, trying to find an altitude without heavy cloud cover. The radioed message said the pilot could not see to orient the plane, which in fact had gone off course and was falling quickly. It hit a hydro wire, burst into flames, and crashed. The three men on board (Harry, the pilot, and a journalist who was dedicated to getting public support for the struggle) were killed. We mourned all three of the crash victims, especially our dear friend. The forewarning Harry had shared with us was a mysterious comfort, but it did not alleviate the pain of his loss.

Jim did not talk about his friend or weep. He simply entered more deeply into his own stillness. I found it impossible to juggle medical school and a husband whose mourning I could not help.

I asked my student counsellor if I could quit. He advised me not to. The answer was to set up sessions with a psychiatrist for us both. We were still in our first year of marriage. Mourning the tragic loss of a friend, juggling the difficulties of a marriage in two cities, coping with a demanding career — these struggles did not provide me with a reason to rest. Luckily, I also had mononucleosis, so the university granted me three weeks of time off. Illness afforded me some desperately needed recovery time.

2

EAST IS THE TIME OF SPRING
AND NEW BEGINNINGS

When I returned to school, I sought alternatives for electives that would take me away from the large teaching hospitals in Hamilton. One was an inner-city clinic with a warm, down-to-earth doctor, Cynthia Carver. I worked in her Toronto office one month in early spring and started to feel human again. I thought maybe I could still be a physician, after all. Under her wise and skilled supervision, I learned basic skills, to give needles, and to see patients on my own.

The second escape route took me to Scotland, to work with midwives for two months later that spring. My father-in-law was of Scottish descent and had legions of smiling, cheery, impossible-to-understand relatives along the whisky trail in northeastern Scotland. So we incorporated a long-overdue holiday with Jim's parents and my work delivering babies at a small cottage hospital outside Edinburgh, in Broxburn, West Lothian. The various cousins, who mostly lived in stone cottages, taught me to drink single malt whisky, a skill I quickly mastered and have retained, with some practice, to this day.

I was delighted to discover I could practise drinking single malt while I was on call. The hospital staff would take supper at the local pub, a smoky room filled with laughter, dart players, and people of all ages, including children with their parents. I would watch as everyone drank "Barmaid's Blush" (lager with Campari), as well as the equally popular lager and lime. This all seemed very civilized. The registrar and senior house officer, as the chief resident and intern were termed, would happily sit, joking with the midwifery students.

I was a strange go-between, a Canadian medical student training primarily under the supervision of the senior midwives. Someone's pager would beep, and we would pay up and troop over to Bangour, the cottage hospital comprised of several portable outbuildings thrown up during the war. The winding road back from the pub traced its way through the psychiatric hospital grounds, stately old brick buildings surrounded by lawns and trees, and ended at Bangour. Each of the portables had a different ward, so we might first go to Labour and Delivery but then have to pop back to our bedroom to collect a stethoscope. If we had to take blood, perhaps to get the patient's blood type and prepare for a possible blood transfusion if a Caesarean section was needed, we would have to bring the sample to another long rectangular building that housed the lab.

The pubs were great, but the hospital canteen was not. Spam fritters should be banned from the planet. Fatty Spam slices, deep-fried so they ooze grease, were Tuesday's inedible fare. Chip butties, another standard, were sandwiches slathered with margarine, with french fries as the filling. The one benefit to this culinary introduction is that they reappeared when I taught at the Liverpool School of Tropical Medicine in the early 1980s. Blood pudding was another delight. At least it was salty.

There was another Canadian at Bangour, Dr. Clare Heffernan, who was doing "a house job," or internship. She was relaxed and walked with easy strides. She had long, wavy dark brown hair and a perpetual smile as we did "blood rounds," taking blood from the women in various stages of pre- or post-delivery. Though midwives could deliver the babies and, in Canada, lab techs could do venipunctures, this was a job in Scotland for doctors and medical students only. I never saw Clare stressed over a patient. She was always cheerful and seemed to know exactly what to do all of the time and was comfortable giving or seeking advice. At her side, I seemed to effortlessly absorb the skills from her that had seemed impossible to learn at Mac.

After our early-morning blood rounds on my first day, there was a delivery. Having only been able to witness three births from a distance in Canada, this would be my first one up close. Brigid, the midwife in charge that day, kindly asked me, "Come on love, do you want to deliver this one? I know you're used to putting the mums up in stirrups. We don't do that. See, here is the wee lassie; she's tiring a bit, but she's just lying in the bed resting between her contractions. When she starts to push, I will stand on one side of the bed and you on the other, and she can push her feet against our sides. When the bairn just pops out, we have the bed beneath the wee thing so it is safely born."

We were both wearing street clothes, with just a green over-gown on our fronts. We did have gloves on and a mask over our face — no sterile cap was needed. I stood on one side and Brigid on the other. Theresa was having her first baby and her husband, Malcolm, was caressing Theresa's face. Brigid smiled encouragingly. "All right, there. Now push, Theresa, push, that's a girl, while I just stretch you a wee bit during the contraction. You're nearly there; I think that last lip of the cervix was taken up that time."

Theresa smiled bravely and pushed again and again.

"So there, Dr. Gretchen, you just get ready like so. Here's the head — just keep your left palm against it so it doesn't come too quickly in case the cord is wrapped around the babe's neck, and check for that with your right forefinger. There you are then! The head is out, and feel there. Ah, that's just great, no cord. Okay, now, next push! — the babe will just pop out. Oh, here she is, easy now. Just let her gently onto the bed. Oh, listen to her cry! And now we have the clamps for the cord. That's it, well done. Now you cut the cord just there, perfect, and we wrap the babe like this and over to mum! Theresa, you can put the babe to the breast, and that will help you with stopping the bleeding and getting out the afterbirth."

The new parents were both a little teary but smiling hugely. Theresa started to suckle the baby. Brigid turned back to me. "Now, here we are. We watch for the lengthening of the cord and then pull gently down. That's it. Controlled traction, there you go. Just let the placenta pop into this dish. That's it. Then you check and make sure it's complete, and nothing has been left inside her. Well done! Your first birth in Scotland! Now off you go to make tea and toast for the mum."

I loved what I was doing, and with every phone call, I would jump quickly out of bed and run over to Labour and Delivery for another birth. I loved being in Scotland, farther north than anywhere I'd been; the sun would already be hinting its arrival at four in the morning, its streaky pink shadows warming up the night sky while a cool wind teased my hair. Sometimes I did the delivery; sometimes, if a midwifery student "caught" the baby, I would do the stitching up afterward if needed. Only then would we put the mother up in stirrups, and that was after we had made tea and toast for her and any family members with her.

I grew to love tea and toast. If we had a Caesarean section late at night, after the delivery we would all sit down at a big refectory table for tea and toast — six or eight of us, the senior obstetrician and chief registrar who had done the surgical birth, the midwives who had assisted in the O.R., and the students. I would stroll back across the grass as the sun came up to try to catch at least an hour or two of sleep before the day began and rejoice in being alive.

3

TRUE HOME IN THE SPIRIT

YOU LIVE ON EARTH ONLY FOR A FEW SHORT YEARS
WHICH YOU CALL AN INCARNATION,
AND THEN YOU LEAVE YOUR BODY AS AN OUTWORN DRESS
AND GO FOR REFRESHMENT TO YOUR TRUE HOME IN THE SPIRIT.
— *WHITE EAGLE*

I returned from Scotland rejuvenated. I had been working there for two months, with a week's holiday to start, and Jim had spent a week with me in the midwifery student residence. Though the constant pages in the night had not done much for our stressed marriage, I had a stronger sense of where I could find a place for myself in medicine. After finishing at McMaster, I went on to complete my medical training with one year of interning at St. Joseph's Hospital in Toronto.

I was able to get a rare long weekend off from my internship in the winter to travel with Jim from Toronto to Bear Island. This is an Ojibwe community on Lake Temagami, north of North Bay. Like Lake Temiskaming to the north, Temagami's name also comes from the Anishinaabe word for deep water. Both lakes have huge round holes carved out by glacier movements, several hundred feet deep and a hundred feet or so in diameter.

Our journey involved a seven-hour drive, followed by a half hour on the frozen lake by Ski-Doo. Jim had been asked to work exclusively for the Temagami Indian Band at Bear Island, to help them with their land claim, under the leadership of Chief Gary Potts. Money had been found from a coalition of churches (Protestant, Lutheran, United, Roman Catholic, Anglican — PLURA) as part of their social justice mandate in support of Indigenous people to pay a modest stipend for Jim. Jim's goal for the trip was to start organizing the historical materials required to help the band prepare their case for court.

I wanted to spend as much time up north as I could. I needed to see how my life might evolve: Could I practise medicine there? How would I adapt to life with no running water, a limited social circle, and no professional colleagues?

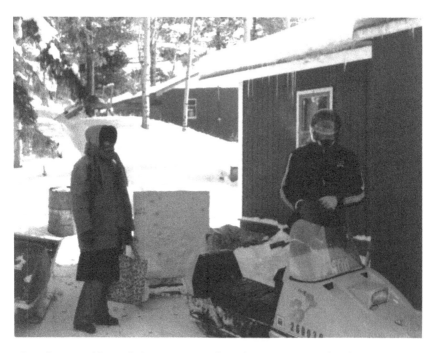

Gretchen Roedde and Gary Potts with a Ski-Doo, Bear Island, Lake Temagami, 1975.

Gary and his wife, Doreen, met us with their snowmobile, which towed a wooden box sled, at the end of the mine road (Lake Temagami Access Road, named after a now long-closed mine on the lake). We had arrived in thick winter clothing — borrowed parkas and snow pants and large Ski-Doo boots. Doreen was wearing a helmet over her long black hair and a zip-up Ski-Doo suit.

Gary joked as he loaded us onto the bare boards of the sled. Doreen slid in behind him on the machine and we roared off, bumping behind them over the frozen lake on the "tree road" — a clear path of solid ice marked with Christmas trees — all the way to Bear Island. We spent four days at their home, sharing meals of bear, pickerel, moose, partridge, beaver, and rabbit.

Jim and Gary worked at the band office, as Jim outlined the plan to interview the Elders in order to make a genealogy chart that would show the link to the current inhabitants, proving occupation of the same geographic area in 1763. The Royal Proclamation of that year stipulated that the "settler governments" had to make treaties with the First Nations for any land transfer to be legal. The Teme-Augama Anishnabai, or Deep Water People, never signed such an agreement, so the community was laying claim to their traditional lands.

While the men worked out how the historical evidence would be gathered and what records would be needed from the Jesuit, Oblate, and Hudson's Bay Company archives, Doreen and I compared notes on looking after sick people. As the Community Health Representative, she had some training in health education but limited clinical skills.

"I don't know how to use a stethoscope to listen to the heart, or wheezing, or pneumonia. I can't take a blood pressure. Maybe you could teach me?"

She worked out of her home, as well as in a small upstairs room near the police station. She explained about the many diabetics in the community, the drunken parties that worried her, and the girls who got pregnant young. "Could we work together on these problems?" she asked shyly.

I said I would help her when we came back in the summer and that I would be relying on her to teach me. I had some medical skills, but she lived in this environment that was so new to me, and she knew the community intimately. I felt so young compared to Doreen. She had five kids; I had none. I was in my early twenties, she in her early forties.

"I want to take you home visiting," said Doreen, who then proceeded to load me up with my parka and scarf into the wooden sled behind the Ski-Doo. "There's just a few people I like to check up on."

There was a huge growl as the engine caught, and the sled swayed side to side as we bounced along the tree trail. Our first stop was to Angenique "just to see how she is getting on. She's one of our Elders."

"Hey, Angenique, how are you?" hallooed Doreen from the front door.

"Oh, I am okay. Just my sore joints. I am drinking wintergreen berry tea. That helps. Good for any kind of rheumatism."

And I did know this was true, that the methyl salicylate in the leaves was an anti-inflammatory painkiller.

One visit led to the next: a young single mom with a new baby; someone coming down off the DTs (delirium tremens, or alcohol withdrawal); spouses who had been involved in a drunken fight, knives included. By the end of that long winter weekend, the cold still chilling me through my Ski-Doo suit, I felt my spirit shift. I had grown up on Toronto Island and knew about cold, icy winters and boat travel. I knew we were about to embark on a grand adventure; this was going to be a truly life-altering decision that was going to be worth giving up the residencies in several specialties I had been offered — family medicine, obstetrics, pediatrics, surgery, psychiatry.

We moved to Lake Temagami at the end of June 1978, and I began a new kind of medical practice. It was a very new way of life in many ways: we had an outhouse, limited (if any) electricity, no running water, and a family income of under ten thousand dollars a year.

It was a glorious day when we arrived; June is still late spring up north. My brave smile hid my worry. I did not know about wood heat, outhouses, or having no phone and only two friends, Gary and Doreen. As we moved the various bags and boxes into the boat, Doreen caught my nervous frown.

"Don't worry. We'll be here to help you. I've raised five kids here. I went as far as grade seven, but my kids went on to high school. I know you've been to university, but you're going to need a lot of teaching! You don't even have kids yet, so you're really more like a kid, not a grown woman. But I'm sure we can help you make out okay! We'll show you how to haul water, heat it on the stove, and store your frozen meat and fish in a *wanagin*, a wooden box that you keep outside your home. It gets to forty degrees below zero, so you'll have your very own freezer! So enjoy summer; it won't last long!"

Doreen gave a shy smile, showed me where to sit in the boat, and told me to get a jacket on as the wind and wet spray would be cold. She nodded to Gary. He could go ahead and start the boat. He and Jim were sitting up front, and I sat back, somewhat dazed, as the sun sparkled on the dark blue water of Lake Temagami.

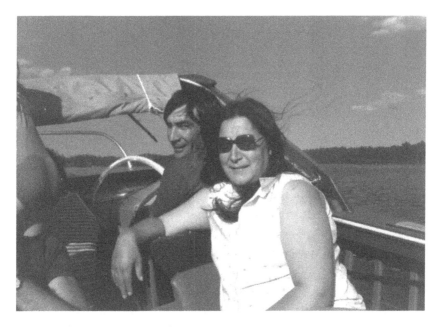

Gary and Doreen Potts, Lake Temagami, 1978.

Lake Temagami has few cottages. Development has been halted to protect the pure water of the lake. The water is so pure that you can drink it right from the lake. More than thirty-five years later, this is still true.

I was busy watching the buoys, green and red markers guiding us to deep water and away from shallows or rocky outcrops. There are very few maples (this area is the northern limit for maples), but one island had a stand of them, a sugar bush. It was used to provide many families with several gallons of syrup a year when Gary and Doreen were young; at the time we arrived, only a couple of families tapped a tree or two.

Driving by boat is a thrilling experience: the motor growls, and there is a faint smell of fuel; the lake is studded with islands covered with red and white pines as well as white poplar and birch; and the boat swerves merrily from side to side, spraying you with clean-tasting water.

Gary and Doreen then drove us by boat to the first of three cabins we would call home for the next two years, all paid for by the band (the most expensive for seventy dollars a month). Our new chapter had begun.

———

The first weeks after our arrival were fairly easy, with bright, sunny days and wide-open, star-filled skies at night. My first patient was Gary's brother Wayne's cat, who needed stitches removed. I must have done okay with her, because a week later Gary drove over in the boat with his niece, who had gotten a fish hook stuck in her leg.

"I know what to do, Gretchen. I'll push the hook through, but it's in deep and it will hurt her too much. You put in the freezing and maybe get some of that antiseptic stuff you brought up with you."

So we worked together. I cleansed the wound with iodine and injected some local anesthetic, and Gary clamped the needle driver over the fish hook so he could push it all the way through and out of the skin.

"Thanks," said Gary simply, helping his niece back into the boat to drive her home.

Doreen came by the next day to thank me again and said maybe I could come with her to do some more home visiting, as we had done previously in the winter.

"People are a bit curious about you. They know that Jim is working for the land claim, so you're probably okay, too. We have a couple of doctors who have cottages on the lake, but we don't like to bother them too much unless someone is real sick. But you're going to be living here all year round. I want you to get to know some of the Elders, like Angenique, who can teach you a lot of the old medicines."

This time Doreen loaded me into an open steel boat. An open boat has no protection from spray, and I got wetter and colder as the minutes passed. Twenty minutes later, I was feeling very chilled as we travelled by Temagami Island, with its maple cover, toward Bear Island. The sky was a deep royal blue, and puffy clouds scudded high overhead. The water was a darker blue, almost slate. From a distance, Bear Island looked to be mostly covered with grey-green trees, but as we got closer we could see small homes nestled between the trees and winding paths leading up from the water. The haunting calls of two loons echoed across the water.

We steered the boat over to the dock down by the band office and recreation centre. Then I saw small moving people, most wearing blue jeans and T-shirts, calling out to each other and laughing. After docking the boat, Doreen and I went up a red pine needle–strewn path to old Angenique's, welcomed along the way by small grey-brown and white birds chirping "chick a dee dee dee," and I thrilled to hear this joyful chattering in the midst of the sounds of a slight wind in the high branches.

Doreen called in after knocking at the front door. "Hey there, Angenique, I've got someone here to see you. She met you last winter. She's a new Medicine Woman, and I told her you were an old one! Huh! What do you think of that?"

"Well, I'm not too old, not yet anyway," said Angenique, smiling. She looked to be in her late seventies. "But sure, I can tell her about how we used to do things."

Once Doreen had made the introduction, I could come on my own and learn about wintergreen berry tea for pain or fever. I could also make poultices from plantain leaves to treat skin problems. Angenique, in turn, introduced me to "Little Mary," whose kids were grown but who had delivered babies when she was a young woman.

"Oh, it wasn't hard. My mom taught me. I'd get water boiling on the woodstove and wash my hands real careful. I'd boil the string to tie the cord and a knife to cut the cord. It was harder in the winter to keep those new babies warm, but we managed. Sometimes we'd put goose grease on the babies' chests and a rabbit fur next to the skin. We've lived in the bush here for hundreds, maybe thousands of years. We still remember some of the old ways. One time at breakup, a woman in the community started to hemorrhage after she gave birth. I was able to find a special plant medicine for her poking up through the snow. I was able to get the bleeding to stop."

It was hard for me to shift gears after my intense medical training. I was trying to patch together meaning from a limited caseload, some public health initiatives, learning to recognize the constellations like Orion and the Big Dipper, and trying out moose recipes. One day Jim came home after I had prepared a moose steak dinner with a Cumberland sauce. He rushed in, grabbed some papers, and said he wasn't staying.

"But I've been cooking all day! Just try this."

"No, Gary is waiting for me. I have to go."

I turned my head to hide my disappointment. This would not be the time to mention "what I had given up for his work." Even as a rant it was untrue; I had chosen to come here, and I was learning so much. And the reality of having no phone is that you can't give advance notice that you are cancelling dinner. Jim's role was more defined. But we were living different lives. I saw more of the community's pain and need for healing, and I craved human contact separate from work. I needed an evening to have supper with my husband. Jim grabbed his papers and left. Fighting back tears, I opened my book of Ojibwe words and phrases: "*Makwa* — Bear. *Wabi Makwa* — White bear. *Ningotaaj* — I am afraid. *Ningashkendam* — I am sad. *Waawaate* — Northern lights," and poured myself the first of several glasses of Côtes du Rhône red.

While PLURA was providing a salary for Jim, the community of Bear Island was responsible for providing us with shelter. The band had "borrowed" two different unused cabins on nearby vacation properties — one we had stayed in for the summer and the second for the fall — both not winterized. That winter, we had moved into our third home, located on island 762, owned by Dick and Vicki Grant. Dick was a Toronto transplant who was a lawyer and had sailed around Toronto Island when he was a student. Vicki, a stunning six-foot beauty (Dick, himself, was six feet three), was a McKenzie from Bear Island. They met when Dick, a recent law school grad, took a year off to run a canoe camp in Temagami. They lived with Vicki's four-year-old son, Fabe, in "the big house down the hill," and we lived above Dick's shop in three rooms heated by a wood fire, with no running water. Unlike the previous cabins, we could stay on island 762 all winter, as long as we kept the woodstove going.

When you live in a city, the friends you choose tend to be similar to yourself — same education, profession, or political preferences. In smaller communities, one's neighbours and friends can come from more varied walks of life. We were now living on a very small island, and our only neighbours were Dick, Vicki, and Fabe. Bear Island was twenty minutes away by boat, and its population was comprised of a few hundred First Nations people. Most of the islands on the lake were uninhabited, but a few had cottages for visiting Americans in the summer. Only a handful of white people lived on the lake year-round.

I wasn't sure it would work for us. As we didn't know how long we would be working with the Bear Island community, I was uncertain how deeply to put down roots. There were now three next-door neighbours, one a small child. What did I, a lifelong New Democrat, have in common with an Upper Canada College–educated Tory? Vicki would be my closest woman friend geographically. What if we didn't get along?

We may have had little in common, but it would be our neighbour Vicki who taught me how to drive a steel boat and then, in winter, a Ski-Doo, and, in between, how to juggle both. During the intense weeks of late fall, you drive the Ski-Doo while towing the boat, then switch to driving the boat with the Ski-Doo in it when you reach a stretch of open water. Vicki was very important in helping me feel grounded. For months I was a bit disoriented. My routine had been completely disrupted, I had no familiar role as a doctor, and I was displaced from the bustling city of Toronto to an isolated island on a lake with only a couple of hundred people. It took many months for me to start to feel as though this was my true home and not some borrowed life.

I loved looking out our large front windows at the red pines and, beyond them, the slate-blue waters of Lake Temagami. I kept the pale green plywood floors scrubbed clean. I could hear the sound of the large pileated woodpecker outside our bedroom window. It was a hard life, though. There were not many white people who supported the land claim, which was isolating, or many who lived on the lake year-round; and we were very urban academics lacking practical skills to live in the bush. As a doctor, I also had certain boundaries with the community: women patients would come by boat to our island with bruised thighs and black eyes from beatings — the perpetrators being members of the community where Jim worked. It is hard to socialize when you are too painfully aware of your neighbours' personal problems. Further complicating matters, Jim and I had different perspectives on how to help. I would be upset by cases of family incest or domestic violence and seek more female leadership in the community and more attention to social problems. He would see the problem as the legacy of the residential schools and insist that the land claim was the solution. We could not afford to fight about these issues. On one occasion, a lawyer colleague was defending a First Nations adolescent from Manitoulin Island who'd been charged with incest with his sister. "I don't know why the girl is making such a big deal about this. It's cultural," the lawyer said. Jim had nodded; I had remained silent instead of defending the brave girl. I often felt unable to voice an opinion. As I later discovered in my work in Third World countries, gender-based violence was common, especially if alcohol was involved. In First Nations and the developing world, male leaders were known to beat their wives when they were drinking — yet had outstanding leadership skills when fighting with the wealthy world for the rights of poor communities. As an outlet for the many unsaid differences of opinion threatening to boil over, Jim and I would play fiercely competitive card games in the evenings, barely keeping divorce at bay.

My spirit felt freer without the constant pressure of long days and nights in a city hospital. I had gotten used to the sound of a motorboat (or Ski-Doo in winter) roaring toward my home — a family member or friend coming to tell me that someone was sick. Sometimes I travelled to see the sick patient if they were too ill to come to me. I once sent a man with a knife wound two hours by boat and road to the hospital because I was worried the puncture was too close to the kidney. Some conditions I could treat with my simple stock of antibiotics. On many occasions when it was too unsafe to travel, I relied on Gary, Doreen, and the family of patients to accurately describe what had happened. One winter night, when the weather was too bad for me to venture back out, I sent along some narcotics for an older woman to help with the pain of her broken hip. "She'll have to go out tomorrow and meet the ambulance at the mine road to get to hospital, but these Demerol pills will help her tonight."

Some illnesses did not get better; sometimes it was just time for an Elder to leave this life. This was in contrast to the harried activity and testing I had seen in medical school. People who live in the bush, in isolated or extreme conditions, know that life is really part of the wheel: that it can be dangerous; that all animals, including us, die. The Bear Island community was now teaching me about everyday life and death.

During freeze-up we could not travel at all. Jim and I and Vicki spent those two weeks together, confined to island 762. That was when I discovered I was pregnant, news which I shared excitedly with Vicki, who was three months along in her second pregnancy.

Once we could travel again, Jim and Vicki would travel by Ski-Doo on the tree road over to Bear Island to work. I would go over a couple of days a week to see patients, either with Doreen or with Little Mary's daughter, Mae, who was a nurse, if she was visiting. One day there was a two-year-old child sick with pneumonia. I had antibiotics, but we needed someone to look after the child because the parents were partying. Doreen, Mae, and I looked around the community and found a suitable, quiet home with no smoking or drinking. We "volunteered" the mature couple who lived there to nurse the child back to health for a week. I realized the community was part of our health team, just as I, as a medical doctor, was part of their community.

At home, I kept busy with household chores and had started to write curriculum for a Community Health Representative program with Treaty No. 9. One day, Jim, Vicki, and Fabe travelled in convoy on their way back from Bear Island to island 762. Vicki was on her Ski-Doo, with Fabe on the seat behind her. Jim was following behind on a second Ski-Doo. About halfway to island 762, they approached Chimo Island. Vicki hit a patch of weak ice and went through. She quickly went into rescue mode to lift Fabe off the Ski-Doo, and, luckily, she was able to push Fabe to safety. Jim, following in the second machine, slowed it to a stop. He then edged over to pull Vicki out of the freezing water and help Fabe up onto the strong ice. He managed to get them both to safety and over to the home of our friends Ray and Anne, who lived on Chimo Island. Ray and Anne provided warm baths and dry clothes for Vicki and Fabe before Ray then drove them home, with Jim following. The Ski-Doo that Vicki had been driving was never found.

Friends and neighbours grow close when survival is so basic. Rod and Linda, married teachers on the island across from ours, often had to help us out of the slush when our Ski-Doo got stuck. They also offered the loan of a washing machine and bathtub when hauling water and heating it up on the stove got too tough.

Vicki's loud laugh comforted me as I worried my way through my first pregnancy. By late spring, Vicki was my best friend. Once, we were in her living room, which had huge windows that overlooked the lake and smelled reassuringly of burning birch from their woodstove. I had sat unusually still for a whole day as Vicki taught me to make small moccasins for my baby. Vicki was guiding me in my stitching of the deerskin and also proudly pointing out the beautifully beaded *tikinagan* (cradle board) she had made to welcome her own baby, who was soon to come into the world. As we sat together, both of us hugely round, I

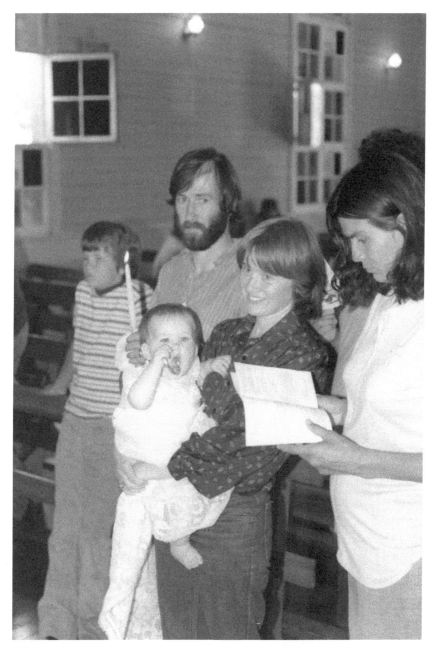

Anna's baptism, with her parents (centre) and godmother, Vicki McKenzie Grant (right), Bear Island, Lake Temagami, 1979.

looked over at her. I knew she was a Catholic, as we had been to Mass at Bear Island, and I'd accompanied her to the mine road to pick up Father Fisher, to bring him to Mass. I was a bit hesitant as I asked her, "Vicki? When my baby is born, will you be the godmother?"

"Sure, Gretch!" Vicki chuckled and gave me a huge smile. "I will just love that."

Vicki knew more about the traditional skills than most other women her age. When she was a newborn, her mom, Laura, had given Vicki to Laura's own mom (Vicki's grandmother). As a result, Vicki had learned how to speak Ojibwe, make moccasins, concoct various traditional medicines, and many other things that Elders like her grandmother still knew. Parents often handed over their children to the grandparents, in part to preserve the traditions that they themselves were forgetting.

Caring for new life was also healing. Laura had just found it too sad to look after her baby girl after giving birth to five boys, because there had once been another daughter who had died young, and Vicki reminded her mother of that loss. When Laura had Vicki, Laura's own mom had just lost a grown son, who had been struck and killed by a falling tree. So Laura sent Vicki to her mom, to comfort her after the loss of her own child. That gave Laura some time to remember and mourn her other child without being reminded by the newborn.

That pattern of grandmothers caring for grandchildren was repeated when Vicki had her first child, Fabe, who was born when Vicki was still a teenager. Laura, in turn, raised him when he was young so Vicki could go to school. Just as Vicki's ties to her maternal grandmother were strong, Fabe and his grandmother had a special bond and were very close.

The two sat together at the funeral for Fabe's great-grandfather. The smell of steam and sweat rose off the wet clothes of the mourners, who stood or sat near the grieving family. Elders sat in worn, mismatched easy chairs so they could stretch their legs out. At least half a dozen people had stayed with the family for days and nights at a time for the wake before the funeral Mass.

My gumboots squeaked as I shook off the remains of the path at the door. The rhythmic chanting of "Hail Mary, full of grace" drifted out the window to those waiting, smoking on the porch. The funeral Mass for Vicki's grandfather, Old Donald McKenzie, was about to begin.

It was the end of my first year on the lake — and my first funeral. I was moved by how the Deep Water People pulled together when there was a death. As the Hail Mary echoed through the room and beyond, everyone's voices in unison, I could feel how connected everyone was, though often it was the broken pieces I had to support.

I did not make eye contact with anyone. Some of the pieces that felt broken to me were in the room. The day before, I had been asked by Linda, the teacher living on the neighbouring island, to visit the public school to see two young girls. That morning, before the funeral, I had brought my pregnancy testing kit to the school. Bear Island is the largest community on Lake Temagami and hosts a one-room schoolhouse for students, mostly Indigenous, from junior kindergarten to grade eight. I tried to see each of two young girls discreetly and get them to give me a urine specimen. One was in grade seven, one in grade eight. Linda and I sat with each girl one at a time and explained that she was pregnant. I told Linda that I would go with the girls at lunch to help them break the news to their loved ones. That had been very difficult, and I was now avoiding Linda's eyes and those of the two girls, who were also at the funeral.

When Jim and I got home that night, we talked. "It's tough to see such young girls get pregnant!" I exclaimed.

In a calm voice, he replied, "Getting pregnant young is a cultural tradition. In the past, if they were too young to look after the babies, there'd always be others who'd formally or informally adopt the kids. What's changed is that more of the Elders are drinking, so there are fewer adults who are responsible enough to be good adoptive parents."

I was still furious. One of the girls had become pregnant by a much older man. I knew that both Jim and I were from a culture different from Bear Island's, but our inherent biases about gender were different. Alcohol was a factor in the high rates of teen pregnancy and sexually transmitted diseases, but so too was the low status of women. I angrily went to bed, unspoken arguments on my mind.

That spring, the Bear Island schoolkids did a project where they made pictures about what they were seeing at home: images of parents fighting, fallen on the ground, passed out; pictures with lots of booze on the table; drawings of kids crying alone in their rooms as their parents partied. Linda called me over to look through them.

As an educated white woman from a middle-class home, Linda found it hard to understand the reality her students faced. "Sometimes the kids come in to school, and there has been fighting through the night. We often bring them to our place for a day or two when things at home get too crazy. You've seen the fighting; it can get really bad. Any idea what we can do?"

I talked to the Chief and Council. Maybe it was time to try to do more about the drinking. Maybe the drinkers themselves were not ready, but the families were ready to learn more about how they could limit the damage it was doing to their kids and to themselves. At that point, I had a little more credibility in the community than when I had arrived. I was no longer a girl and would have a baby later that summer. Vicki was my mentor and teacher. Her newborn, McKenzie, had arrived in May, weighing around ten pounds, and she was breastfeeding. Our neighbour Linda was also pregnant, due in June. So by that June of 1979, I had a good idea what was in store for me. I thought I should take advantage of still being able to travel fairly easily.

I checked out St. Joseph's programs for alcohol abuse in North Bay, an hour and a half south by road after a half-hour boat ride. St. Jo's had a one-month session for the drinkers and a one-week course for affected family members. I called up the nuns who ran the centre and asked if I could attend for a week and participate in both. I needed to know if the courses would be okay for the community members. Would they be too religious, too patronizing? I wasn't going to send anyone to St. Jo's if I didn't know what they would experience. The high rate of substance abuse among First Nations people is partly related to the downside of cultural domination by Canadians and our institutions. We made their spiritual leaders illegal, moved people off their large traditional lands and into small communities, and removed children from their families for forced education and often brutal foster care. Ripped away from culture, family, religion, and language, these kids were too often sexually or physically abused by white clergy and/or foster parents. I needed to ensure that my patients would not end up being subjected to more harmful treatments by white people.

Jim drove me down to North Bay, hugged me goodbye, and went on to do some provisioning. He had included Tia Maria, bags of milk, and boxes of bran flakes on the shopping list — all favourites of mine during my pregnancy. He was also going to find me some murder mysteries — his way of supplying constant bibliotherapy sedatives for me. I carried a small bag on wheels, with clothing to last me a week. The other participants and facilitators — former priests and practising nuns — joked about whether they would have to deliver me. No subtle bump mid-abdomen for me. Only six and a half months along, I looked like I was having twins — today. My Kmart maternity panels stretched in the cheap corduroy slacks, and I wore a loose lilac blouse. While I had explained that I was there to help the Bear Island community, I had to participate as well. I had to share my own hard times when the others divulged what had led them to drink. I could not hide behind being a doctor. I realized it was good to discover how painful self-discovery can be, especially if I was going to send patients here. I had my own family history of substance abuse. The group helped me understand that working a hundred hours a week, as I had done in my years of medical training, could be its own form of addiction, only one that gets rewarded. I opted against telling them that Tia Maria and milk was my current drink of choice; after all, pregnant women need calcium, right? Many of the thirty residential patients had been referred by the courts for alcohol addiction treatment after DUIs (driving under the influence) or drunken assaults. Others had been told by spouses to get help, *or else*. The centre was non-judgmental and truly committed to helping people, but the counsellors would not tolerate anyone's bullshit.

I thought the centre would be helpful for the people of Bear Island, whether they were the drinkers themselves or the family who loved them. The one-week program had many insights regarding how family members can sabotage a drinker's attempts at recovery. The non-drinker is in a position of power, because the drinker keeps messing up. Once the alcoholic starts to recover and act more responsibly, the power position shifts. Sometimes the family then sabotages the drinker's efforts to get sober, to restore the power balance back in favour of the non-drinkers. Oftentimes it is the anxiety level of the non-drinker, worriedly waiting for the drinker to fall off the wagon again. So they needle the drinker to get them to start drinking sooner rather than later — just to get it over with. These were all helpful reflections to understand the dance of co-dependency and how alcoholism is a disease affecting the whole family or community. I thought the one-week family program would help at least the people in the community living with alcoholics.

The week sped by. Late Friday afternoon, it was time to leave North Bay and get back to Bear Island. I would take the bus to Temagami, and Gary would pick me up and drive us down the mine road. After the drive, the rest of the trip home would be five miles by boat to island 762, where Jim was waiting.

It was a rough night for driving. The wind was picking up and howling in the trees as I waited at the bus stop in Temagami. Gary's mud-splattered truck came to a stop; he waved me in with a cheery grin. "You better not have that baby tonight!" he said, laughing.

He had on a Bear Island Braves ball team T-shirt and wore a ball cap over his black hair. His truck was loaded up with plastic bags and boxes of groceries. I squeezed into the passenger seat. As we lurched along the mine road, gravel blew around and pelted the truck as the treetops tossed madly, and rain started to cascade down in sheets. Ten feet ahead of us, a frightened fox almost blew across the road. This did not bode well for the boat ride to come.

When we reached the dock, I gathered up my bag and held it over my head to protect me from the blinding rain. Gary steadied the boat as it swung wildly in the waves and loaded it with his groceries as I managed to get myself onto a seat. Gary looked up at the sky. "I don't think we can get to 762. The wind is coming against us. Maybe you can stay at Bear Island tonight?"

We took off as waves poured over the sides of the open steel boat, drenching us both. I remembered that Gary's brother had drowned in the deep waters of this same lake on a stormy night. He had been with a woman from Bear Island. Few people at Bear Island can swim. Although I am a strong swimmer, my pregnant state, combined with wind and wild waves and thoughts of those who had died on this very lake, had me worried. The waters of Lake Temagami are nearly four hundred feet deep in places.

As we sped through the churning water, the waves lifted and crashed down in the open steel boat, drenching us and tossing us around crazily. The spray chilled my arms and face, but I had faith in Gary. He had been driving boats since he was a kid. He had not been drinking; I never saw him drink and drive, neither boat nor truck. I was worried about the new life I was carrying, also moving rhythmically inside me, and I wondered how my little family would fare in the harsh weather of our environment. Half an hour later, we poured ourselves out at Gary's dock, cold and wet. My teeth were chattering uncontrollably, my hugely pregnant body made even heavier by my soaked clothing. I felt like a hippo lurching onto land. Though weak and exhausted, I was also triumphant and relieved after such an adrenaline-filled trip home.

Doreen welcomed us with hot partridge soup, her long black hair framing her smiling oval face. There was no phone at island 762, so there was no way I could let Jim know I was okay, but I hoped he wouldn't worry. Gary and Doreen moved Paula, their youngest daughter, onto the couch in the living room, and I slept in her bed, thankfully cradling my pregnant belly, feeling that unborn life moving mysteriously under my cupped hands. As the wind tore through the trees and rain lashed against the roof, the whole house shuddered. I listened in awe until I finally dropped off into a deep sleep.

In the morning, I woke uneasily, disoriented, unsure where I was. "Old Tom Peabody Peabody Peabody" scolded an unseen bird hidden in the red pine boughs above. I dressed slowly, in the clothes from the day before. Shyly, I came into the kitchen to find Doreen boiling water for tea, cooking porridge, and frying bannock. The kids weren't up yet. I could see Paula asleep on the couch. Gary came in from the dock, where he had been getting the boat ready, and we sat down at the breakfast table. Sun streamed in through the windows; a light breeze rippled the curtains. After we had tea and bannock, I gathered up my things. "Thanks for everything, Doreen, the bed, and the breakfast," I said quietly and gave her a quick hug as she stood at the sink; she smiled slightly.

The air was still and cool, and the sky was a soft blue overhead. Gary loaded up the boat and expertly started it with one quick pull. Twenty minutes later, as we pulled up at the back dock at island 762, Jim came down to greet us. "I wasn't worried!" he said. "I knew Gretchen was safe with you!"

He reached over to pick up my bag and gave my cheek a peck. Gary backed the boat out with a happy wave as he prepared to return home.

Jim and I walked up the uneven path, carefully stepping over the roots embedded in the soil, the breeze blowing us the scent of the red pines overhead. *Yes*, I thought, *I am returning home*. Although my own roots are only thinly planted here, this is my path, and I will see where it leads me.

———

A month later, Vicki's mom, Laura, got sick. It was terminal cancer, and it was the first and only time I saw Vicki shaken. "Look after Fabe," she said. I took care of five-year-old Fabian as she went off, carrying her infant son McKenzie to the hospital in North Bay, where her mom was dying.

Fabe took her sudden departure very hard; he was stressed and kept to himself. He often went outside, sat on a fallen log a distance from our place, and cried. He didn't want anyone near him. For the two days Vicki was away, I would bring him snacks to his outside log, and once I could coax him inside, I'd read his favourite books to him. I felt unsure parenting this child. My own child was due in a month, and I felt unsure about that adventure, too. I did not talk about Laura to Fabe. He knew she was very sick, and from the depth of his grief, I think he understood he was losing his surrogate mother, his grandmother. Two days later, Laura died.

When Vicki came to get Fabe, he reached up to her and sniffled. "It's okay, Fabe, shoosh. She is at peace now." Vicki gathered him into her arms, and he buried his face in her coat. "We're going now, over to Bear Island to get everything ready. A bunch of your cousins have come. There'll be lots of kids you can play with. Then we'll go in the boat and get Father Fisher, who is doing her funeral Mass."

I prepared my own way. Laura was a woman who was deeply loved and respected in the community. I knew the death would be a terrible load for the community to bear. On the day of the funeral, I prepared a backpack with a stethoscope, blood pressure cuff, Aspirin, nitroglycerin, Demerol, and Gravol in injection form. I was worried that someone might have a heart attack.

Everyone was gathering at St. Ursula's, a small Catholic church, for the funeral. I walked slowly, making my way down to the back dock, releasing the scent of pine as the needles crunched under my feet. I got into the steel boat and managed to get the motor started after only a couple of pulls on the cord, then drove the five miles to Bear Island, both lulled by the throbbing engine and alert from the cold waves misting my face with their spray. I docked at the landing and made my way up the winding road, then climbed up the steep path to the little white church in the woods to join the mourners.

Light streamed in through the stained glass, and dogs roamed up the central aisle. I sat with Fabe. Laura's husband, Maurice, sat with his daughter and his sons and their wives. The McKenzies are all tall, with wide faces. Maurice shook his head with grief. The church was nearly full; everyone was in their best clothes to say goodbye to Laura. A murmuring hush of gentle voices filled the room. A light breeze filtered through the open door as a few latecomers entered.

Vicki was strong and composed as she spoke of her mother. "We always had other kids staying with us, and Mom could always make

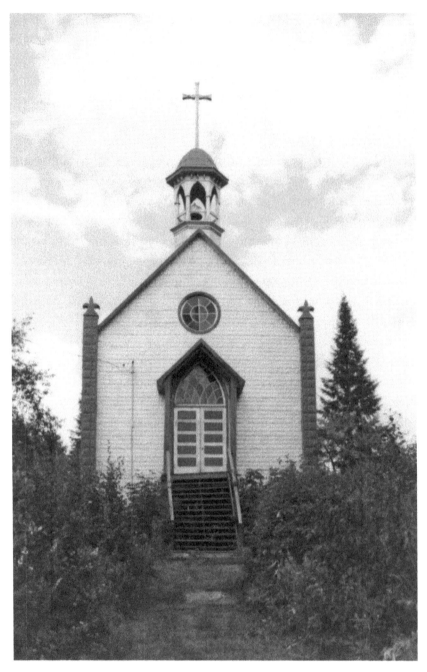

St. Ursula's Roman Catholic Church, Bear Island, Lake Temagami.

room for one more. Somehow she was always in control, and that isn't easy with a house filled with my dad and brothers!"

Father Fisher reminded us of how this good woman had lived a great life of the spirit, always there to help others. "While we mourn her death, we can honour her life by living as she has done."

I had met Laura only a handful of times, but she seemed the image of quiet strength. The funeral Mass included communion, and as each person went up to receive the Host, they placed their hands lightly on the shoulders of Laura's family.

After the service, we filed out of the church and headed down the path and over to the trail that led to the graveyard. All-terrain vehicles roared ahead, transporting those who had trouble walking. The rest of us walked slowly through the woods, passing pale pink wild roses, whose sweet scent wafted over us in the warm light wind of the sunny early afternoon. Occasionally, a rabbit or squirrel would dash across the path and disappear in the woods. The buzzing of bees and a light breeze gently moved the prickly rose briars, releasing more perfume as we arrived at the point of the island where the graveyard was located. The air felt soft on my face.

The men had been out there the day before digging the grave, around which maybe twenty people were now gathered. Vicki and her brothers were first to gather at the hole in the earth. Vicki stood with her family and murmured a prayer, wiped the tears from her eyes, and then threw a few flowers onto the grave. Her brothers Mac and Johnny took turns gently tossing dirt onto Laura's coffin. Vicki's other brothers, sisters-in-law, nieces, and nephews walked to the edge of the grave and tossed in a few more blossoms and handfuls of sand. Then the rest of us took our turns saying our last goodbyes, some of us weeping.

"She was such a good woman. She helped so many of us," murmured Gary Potts.

The community stood together on this lazy summer afternoon with just the sounds of a few birds overhead and a gentle wind in the woods. It was comforting to be gathered together, grieving. The men took turns with shovels to fill the grave. I listened to the hushed voices and watched the flowing tears. I kept glancing back at Maurice, whose face was now contorted with sorrow.

And just as the Bear Island community was joined in grief, moments later it was linked together in reaction to a new crisis. I heard shouting. Someone called my name, "Gretchen, over here, quick!"

It was Linda George, Gary's sister. Her face was creased with alarm. Their dad, old Philip Potts, had fallen to the ground, clutching his chest and groaning. I went to him as quickly as I could, got carefully down on my knees while protecting my pregnant abdomen with one hand, and checked his heart rate — irregular and fast — with the pulse at his wrist. He was gasping, "I feel sick, and it's so heavy in my chest!" He was already starting to slur his words.

"Linda! Help me get this pack off my back. I have medicines in there and a stethoscope!"

Linda pulled the pack from my shoulders. Gary was beside us by this time.

"Here you are, Gretchen." Linda handed me an Aspirin and a nitro-glycerin tab, which I poked into Philip's mouth. She gave me a small bag containing a syringe, needle, and ampoule of Demerol.

"Gary, get help! I think Philip's having a heart attack and maybe a stroke!" I said as I quickly drew up the Demerol and injected it in Philip's right buttock. Then Philip stopped speaking, and his face drooped on one side, the right side of his body motionless.

Gary ran down to a boat at the dock and radioed out for an ambulance to meet us on the other side at the mine road. Linda George kept calling out "Oh no, Dad, no!" She held Philip's hand while her husband, George, helped Gary unhook a spinal board from the dock, one of several placed around the perimeter of the island. They carted it up together a minute later and worked to help load Philip, now unconscious, onto the stretcher.

The grieving McKenzies remained near their mother's grave as the rest of the community sprang into action. Several kids started crying with fear. "What's happening? What's going on? What's wrong with Philip?"

I bent over the stretcher and put my stethoscope on Philip's chest, hearing fast beats skipping around wildly instead of the usual *lubdub lubdub* of two alternating thumps. We started to walk, the men carrying Philip carefully toward the shore. I thought he must have thrown off a clot and had a stroke, judging from the weakness on one side and loss of speech.

It took four people to get Philip into the boat. We roared off, bouncing on the waves, and tried to keep Philip still on the spinal board. Twenty minutes later, we reached the mine road landing. Thankfully, the ambulance was waiting. The paramedics, a woman and a man, rushed to help us dock, then loaded Philip into the back of the ambulance. I rode in the back, Gary up front.

The mine road was pretty tortuous, with rapidly winding turns and a washboard surface of loose gravel. In the back of the ambulance, I stood beside the stretcher, listening to Philip's heart and making sure he was breathing. Ten minutes along, I realized that the combination of my pregnancy and a bumpy ride on a washboard gravel road was going to make vomiting inevitable. I grabbed a metal basin. Gary turned around and asked, "Is it my dad?" No, it was me that was sick.

A couple of minutes later, Philip's heart shuddered and went still. He stopped breathing. I started cardio-pulmonary resuscitation (CPR). Almost immediately, he started to breathe and his heart started again. A moment later, he went into convulsions. I had no medications for seizures, no Valium in any form, and neither did the paramedics. Helplessly, I watched him seize over the next hour and a half to North Bay, while constantly checking to make sure he was still breathing. The ambulance stopped outside the hospital, and we transferred him into the emerg. I reported to the E.R. doc, who had met the ambulance, "He went into atrial fibrillation at a funeral on Bear Island, and then he seemed to have a heart attack and stroke. I gave him Aspirin, nitroglycerin, Demerol, and Gravol. I think he had a brief cardiac arrest and responded to CPR. He has been having seizures since the mine road. Maybe alcohol withdrawal?" Then, as the doctors and nurses took care of Philip, I tried to explain to Gary that the outlook wasn't good. I was pretty sure that Philip wouldn't make it.

There are limits to medicine. Western medications offered Philip drugs for his heart and stroke, but there was very little healing for him at that hospital in North Bay. The doctor told Gary that Philip would live for only a few days, so Gary stayed with Philip for several days and then took him home. "I can help him get well again."

Two weeks later, Gary started the healing process for Philip back on Bear Island. I visited them at home, and Gary explained why he brought his dad home. "They just had him strapped in a chair, drugged up so he could barely lift his head. He just kept drooling. Though there was enough life in him that he would pinch the nurses with his good hand! I had enough. I knew I could look after him better. He would be better in the community than in hospital. They kept talking about putting him in a nursing home, and they said he would never recover. Never talk or walk again. I knew I had to take charge. He's not just another 'drunken Indian' who had a stroke. He is my dad, and I know how I can make him well again."

The whole community helped Philip on this new journey of recovery of mind, body, and spirit. Gary would take him on slow walks through the village. At first, Philip thought it was just after the war.

"Hey now, Philip! You know that's not right!" said Little Mary when Philip and Gary passed her house. "Look at the grey in my hair! No, it is not 1945. It is 1979 now. Nearly summer!"

When Philip came to Laura McKenzie's house, he saw Vicki helping her dad sort through her mom's belongings.

"Hey, Laura!" called Philip, just slightly slurring his speech, the droop on one side of his face showing some improvement.

"Hi there, Philip," said Vicki, quietly. "Yes, we remember Laura too. I'm her daughter, Vicki. She's gone on to her true home in the spirit. She has left us behind; we are still on the journey in the Medicine Wheel. You, too, you crazy idiot! You sure had us worried at Laura's funeral. You always had to be the centre of attention!" Vicki turned to Gary and smiled slightly. "Good for you, Gary, for bringing your dad home. This will be a good healing journey for him with the community, and we'll all help."

∿ 4 ᖡ

EAGLE OVERHEAD

The next month we travelled farther north to visit Christine and Henry, our friends who lived in a close-knit, back-to-the-land community of about forty people. There were no Indigenous people here; this was a gathering of white people, except for a Puerto Rican, "Brown Bob," on the drums, who tended to gather at each other's homes, play music, and share food in the bush near two communities, Charlton and Kenabeek. Huge tables held a potluck supper, mostly tended by women in long skirts or in shorts and T-shirts. Live music, played mostly by men, including Jim, gathered in a circle by the bonfire, filtered over the heads of laughing children. Christine and Henry were an important part of this community. A heritage homestead, which was the main venue for this gathering, was nestled in the woods along Long Lake, which wound like a narrow river for many kilometres.

I asked our friend Kay, who lived in the homestead, how far I could swim. "Just go as far as the open-air amphitheatre. That should be about twenty minutes each way."

I walked down a damp, squelching path to the bank of the river. Mud oozed through moss underfoot. There was no one around, and I had not brought a bathing suit, so I stripped off and slipped into the warm, cloudy water. I kicked off and began a slow modified breast stroke, watching for the landmark. I wondered what Kay meant. An open-air amphitheatre seemed unlikely in the back of beyond.

It was slippery and smooth in the water. A bright blue sky sparkled above me; the grey-green water shimmered around me. A light current moved me along. I did not know how long I had been in the water. Twenty minutes? I saw nothing that looked like an amphitheatre. I was thinking of something like the bleachers at a ball diamond.

High above me, an eagle soared, shadowing my journey. I followed it. I felt like we were tied together, and it was pulling me along through the water. The white head of the bird suggested it was a bald eagle, an endangered species in the region around Lake Temiskaming.

Every now and then, I glanced over at the shore looking for some kind of structure. I had no idea how long I had been in the water. The eagle was still overhead; he and I were journeying. Was he worried how long he could fly? Was he looking for landmarks? I was breathing slowly, calmly, surely. I felt so strong, swimming after the eagle.

That great bird was still overhead, leading me on, when a motorboat with a young couple in it came up beside me. "They've been looking for you! All kinds of people down at the old Muriel Newton-White homestead. They're worried! You've been gone for hours!"

I accepted a large towel and wrapped it around myself to clothe my nakedness. I clambered up into the boat. "Sure, we'll give you a lift back." I looked up; my eagle was still there, watching me. I waved goodbye and made my way back in the boat. Jim and Kay were there on the shore, looking worried. She had been poetic in her description of the amphitheatre — it was just an open field near the homestead. I stood, still chilled, wrapped in my towel. I tried to explain about the eagle, how I had just lost all sense of time.

Walking slowly up the path to the homestead, I remembered a dream I had years earlier — an eagle flying overhead, meeting a mate, and nesting in a cold, wild northern grey and green place. Then years of slow growth and stillness, and one eagle separated from the other and flew south, surrounded by warm tropical colours. Where was I on that journey?

SECTION TWO

SHAWANONG / shah-wuh-noong /
Spirit Keeper of the South

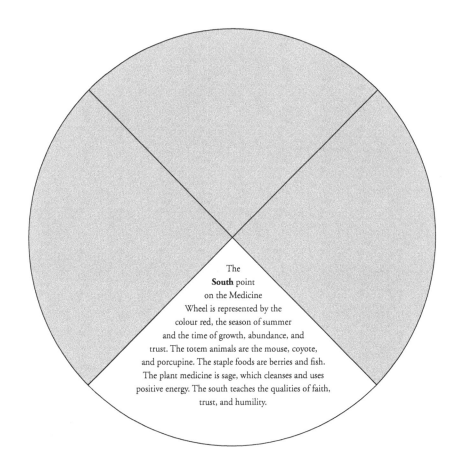

The
South point
on the Medicine
Wheel is represented by the
colour red, the season of summer
and the time of growth, abundance, and
trust. The totem animals are the mouse, coyote,
and porcupine. The staple foods are berries and fish.
The plant medicine is sage, which cleanses and uses
positive energy. The south teaches the qualities of faith,
trust, and humility.

~ 5 ~

BLUEBERRY GIRL

I am burrowed in my blankets. Baby Anna is still sleeping. The ice is talking again. The sky is vastly, deeply quiet and dark. Beyond our cabin, past the red pines that softly surround us, the frozen surface of the lake creaks and groans without moving. In the morning, dressed in jeans and rubber boots and khaki down parka warming my body, I will go down the snowy path, two buckets in my hands. I will walk out onto that ice for six feet to a hole covered by a wooden lid lined with Styrofoam. A chainsaw made that hole three months earlier. Each morning there's a thin crystal layer of ice on the surface. I break it easily with the bottom of my buckets.

My university degrees in anthropology and medicine did not include a component on household water management or on what to do when the fire runs out. They didn't remind me to look at the sky whenever I could. The women in the Bear Island community taught me.

Doreen and the other women gave me a baby shower in the summer of 1979, when I was pregnant with my first baby. After I gave birth, they patiently explained how I should bathe the baby in heated water in a round metal tub.

It takes five buckets of water a day to keep our little home going. I pour the buckets into a large brown plastic garbage pail beneath the sink. We drink the water, wash dishes with it, and heat it up in kettles on the woodstove to fill a tin tub, to bathe the women first — my daughter, Anna, and I (at six months, she just fits in the round tub with me) — then her dad. After we have bathed, I wash our clothes in the soapy water and then use the water that remains to scrub our plywood floors in the three-room cabin: Anna's room, our room, and a living/dining/kitchen area that has a curtained-off section on one wall to hide our porta-potty. This portable toilet has to be emptied frequently and is only for emergencies. The outhouse is down that same snowy path and boasts the luxury of a Styrofoam seat. There is an extension cord that brings limited electricity to our cabin from Dick and Vicki's, farther down the path. We can have an electric light while we play crazy eights, grind coffee beans by kerosene lantern, or listen to recorded music by candlelight.

The ice is still talking. I slowly awake into the eerie half-light that announces morning. My breasts are heavy, leaking milk. I move quietly so as not to wake Jim. I throw on a down vest over my flannel night-gown, put on moccasins, and go to the next room to see Anna.

She is still sleeping, in a hammock suspended from the ceiling to catch whatever warmth we might have in our cool nighttime cabin. She wears a yellow parka and snow pants, which I made from an adult's down vest, and beaded deerskin mukluks. One hand has come out of the parka and its attached mitten, and it has slipped out of the blankets to rest on the mesh of the hammock. The right hand and forearm are mottled with white. My still sleeping, six-month-old daughter, born in blueberry time, has a swollen, frostbitten arm from the cold tempera-ture of our cabin, as the fire had inadvertently gone out.

I call quietly to Jim to relight the woodstove. I gather Anna into my arms. I bring her hand to my warm stomach under my breasts. Carrying her, we move back to bed, and I bundle her under the covers while she nurses, still sleeping. Skin on skin, I re-warm her. As the blood flow returns to her arm, she wakes up crying and shakes her hand in pain.

The ice is still talking. A new sound is added, the growl of a Ski-Doo approaching our island, then roaring up the snowy path. The motor coughs, stops, and a voice shouts for Dr. Gretchen. It is Old Georgie Missabie calling, "Can you help me? My knife slipped earlier this morning when I was filleting pickerel. I bandaged my arm till it was okay to come and see you." He comes into the workshop on the ground floor, then climbs slowly up the short staircase.

I still have Anna on my breast and am warming her body. I throw on another blanket, both for warmth and privacy. I spread out last week's *Globe and Mail* on the kitchen table. From a shelf in Anna's room, I bring out antiseptic, sutures, local anaesthetic, scissors, and a needle driver. I pass sleeping Anna, whose arm is less swollen, to her dad. I pull a lanolin-scented, grey wool fisherman sweater over my flannel nightgown.

George wears a Ski-doo suit over a thick plaid jacket. His face is wide and round, and the skin is slightly pitted with scars. His grin is infectious. "You white guys are crazy! You have a baby in this cold cabin!" He steps into the kitchen from the stairs. His Ski-Doo boots drip melted snow onto the green plywood floor. The woodstove is crackling merrily with the soothing smell of burning birch and has warmed up the bucket of water, its constant companion. I ladle warm water into a dish and dip some clean facecloths into it. I joke a bit with Georgie. "I guess you figure you can trust me to do this, since Wayne Potts brought his cat here to have its stitches out! But it hurts more putting them in. I'll put a little freezing in for you first." I roll up his sleeve and prepare to sew up his arm after washing it in warm water and iodine. I draw up the local anaesthetic and inject it in several places along the wound, which is quite straight and not too long. Georgie winces dramatically and then laughs. "It doesn't really hurt. It's too cold in here to feel anything anyway!" I open up the packet of sutures, black silk, tipped with a curved needle, and place them alongside scissors and the needle driver. It takes six sutures to close the wound. "Georgie, I'll remove the stitches in a week or so. Keep the wound clean with soap and water and any hydrogen peroxide or rubbing alcohol, if you have it, to prevent infection. Come back sooner if it gets reddened or you're worried."

He rolls back his sleeve and zips up his Ski-Doo suit. "And if it gets red I put some rum on it? Or maybe I drink the rum, and then I won't worry if it gets red? Don't worry; I'll be careful to keep it clean. *Meegwetch!* Thank you!" he says, and tramps back down the stairs.

Jim has prepared freshly ground dark roast coffee and is drinking his by the picture window overlooking the lake. Bright natural sunlight streams in the window. He is reading the (Manchester) *Guardian Weekly*, which includes a couple of pages of *Le Monde*, translated into English, and the *Washington Post*. The airmail paper of its pages crackles as he reads, joining the snapping of burning birch logs in the woodstove. The smoky smell of the birch mixes with the dark roast coffee. I add some Tia Maria and milk to my own large pottery mug, which I hold warming my hands. My grandfather drank rum in his morning tea while living on the sailboat he designed; I think the Tia Maria helps with breastfeeding.

"Jim, Anna is going to be okay. Her arm is still mottled, but I don't think the skin will be damaged. It's amazing how quickly the cabin cooled down though. Who knew she has been keeping us all warm by waking in the night for feeds. We're going to need a new plan if she's starting to sleep through the night." Jim gathers up his files for work, and I wave goodbye as he heads off to the band office farther down the lake. I wrap up the stained *Globe and Mail* and toss it in the woodstove, then hold Anna in my arms as I look out the picture window to the snow-covered red pines and the frozen lake beyond. A large pileated woodpecker taps repeatedly on the red pine outside the window. I look down at my baby girl. Her arm is now a normal size but still red. Her intense blue-green eyes seek mine, and she smiles.

———

My blueberry girl. On August 7, 1979, ten days overdue, I was picking blueberries at a sand point, where a forest fire had burnt off the low brush and Labrador tea five years earlier. Every summer since then, sun-warmed blueberries have grown there in abundance. As I stooped to pick the berries, I started to feel the aches that signalled the beginning of my first child's arrival into the world.

The pains continued into the afternoon when I was seeing patients back at the cabin. My last visitor was Linda, whose two-month-old daughter, Sarah, was sick. Linda had noticed me caress my tightening belly and asked about signs of labour. "Have you had any show?" When I admitted I had lost some blood-tinged mucus earlier, before the pains had started, she laughed. "Jim, your wife here is in labour! Get her out to hospital." I was sure I wasn't in labour. I had visions of nurses muttering about a physician who couldn't distinguish between her own false and true labour. But Linda had Jim convinced before she and Sarah headed home. Jim gathered a few days' worth of clothes and simple toiletries into a backpack. We clambered down the path to the back dock and into the steel boat, and we bounced over the waves to the mine road as the sun was setting. After we docked, we made our way up to the parking lot. I felt so heavy, so full of quaking life inside. Suddenly, I was scared.

"This is it!" I said. We packed ourselves into our old car, a Toyota which was on its last legs, and headed off on the hour-long drive to the hospital. We had to keep stopping so that Jim could run to nearby streams and feed the leaking radiator with water. I was rethinking natural childbirth. I likely had several hours to go and was already finding labour difficult. Contractions were coming about every two to three minutes. I was straining, in agonizing pain in the August heat. Once we emerged onto the two-lane highway headed north, we were able to stop at two real restaurants, where Jim ran in to ask for water for our radiator tank. "No problem!" called out the guy in his forties who ran the Chinese restaurant in Temagami. "Good luck!" cried out the grey-haired woman who tended the cash at the Cobalt Truck Stop.

Just before midnight, we arrived at the little hospital in Haileybury. The OB nurse and my Irish GP both checked me and declared I was only fingertip dilated. Nothing, really. Just beginning. Dr. Kelly smiled, patted my hand, and explained in his lilting brogue, "You know I would have come down to Lake Temagami to deliver you, but maybe you were right to come here. That is a big baby, and the head is still high. We'll see how you get on through the night. Try to rest. I'll check you in the morning, and the nurse can call me if things start to move more quickly." Jim spent the night with friends in the next town, New Liskeard.

I laboured hard all night, with no progress by the morning. Dr. Kelly came in to do his morning rounds just as Jim arrived. "The head is still high, so I won't break your waters now. I think you're going to need an oxytocin drip to get things moving. And you're already having a lot of pain. You're going to need some help. You're lucky. We have a new GP who has been working in Australia and does anaesthetics. He'll give you an epidural. I know you trained with midwives in Scotland, and you wanted a simple delivery. But you're already too tired, and we have many more hours to go."

Once the epidural had been put in, I was no longer the anguished woman writhing in pain and occasionally vomiting. From eight in the morning till four in the afternoon, I was pain-free and chatting with Jim. But I had no sensation so could not respond when I was fully dilated. Dr. Kelly was worried, as there had been meconium staining showing that the baby was in trouble, but I could not push. "I'll have to pull the baby out with forceps," he said.

With Jim dressed in greens and caressing my shoulders, Dr. Kelly delivered Anna, who weighed nine pounds, four ounces. I had lost a litre of blood, and Dr. Kelly ordered an intravenous (IV) transfusion of blood. After being transferred to my room and having the blood transfused, I was drinking well, so the IV was discontinued. But the long labour and rough delivery had taken its toll. I felt faint, dizzy, and exhausted. Jim was holding Anna by the bed when I cried out, "I think I'm going into shock!" He shouted for the nurse, who got an IV started again and lowered the head of the bed. I responded well to the treatment but was still weak.

I was also culturally confused. Hours earlier I had been on an island with no running water. Now I was in a small hospital with "medical supports" such as forceps, epidural, other painkillers, oxytocin to help a stalled delivery, fetal and labour monitoring equipment, blood transfusions, and a strong team of nurses and doctors.

Having lost out on my plan to have a natural delivery, I was not going to miss out on breastfeeding. I told the nurses not to give Anna any sugar and water or formula supplements. Colostrum, the fluid which flows before breast milk, is not high in calories. The following day, when Anna was brought in for me to feed, I could not wake her up, even if I rubbed hard on her breastbone, which is a way to rouse someone from a coma. I called out to the nurses, knowing Anna's blood sugar was low, and we quickly needed the sugar and water I'd initially refused to bring her out of the hypoglycemic coma.

———

Three days later, Jim drove us back to our island in that open steel boat, in a rainstorm, against relentless waves. I held our baby girl under my yellow rain slicker, my smallest finger in her mouth to make sure she was sucking and still breathing under all my clothing. When we arrived at the front dock of island 762, Vicki, Anna's Ojibwe godmother, laughed, "You crazy white people! Even Indians wouldn't bring a baby home in this weather!" To have waited for better weather would have meant imposing on the kindness of our friends who lived in town with running water and electricity. In my mind, to have rested longer would have been a sign of weakness. I would be strong for my adored blueberry girl, holding her in my arms on the crashing waves of Lake Temagami.

∽ 6 ᵔ

LEARNING TO TRUST

The room smelled of dirty boots. I looked around at a dozen Ski-Doo suits unzipped to mid-chest. Traces of cigarette smoke wafted from the damp clothes. There were fourteen of us: one white woman doctor and thirteen Cree people from Moose Factory and up the James Bay coast. It would take the work of each person, and all of us together, over the course of one week to create one hundred new Cree words.

Those precious words were to become the basis of a Cree-English medical dictionary, to help to explain symptoms and illnesses to patients who'd flown to the hospitals in Moose Factory or Timmins and spoke no English. It would help Cree patients to feel more at home if their health workers could speak even a few words of their language.

We were in the Ojibwe-Cree Cultural Centre in Timmins. I had arranged for a neighbour on the lake to babysit and had come up on the train from Temagami. In the large classroom, one clean-shaven trapper had brought butchered meat parts and was carefully laying them on a plastic sheet on the table. Greg Spence and his brother Alex acted as translators.

"See, this is the moose liver," said the trapper. "Is there a part like this in the human body? What does it do?" Greg translated the Cree for me, and he talked back and forth with the trapper to make sure he had faithfully understood and translated the trapper's comments correctly. I looked over at the liver. What does it do? What is important to know? I tried to think of what might be relevant for patients.

Nodding, I tried to explain in English, looking carefully at Alex, who would translate my words. "You see it is very bloody? The liver filters the blood. If you take medicines, like Tylenol, it is processed in the liver, or *kiskon(a)*.

Alcohol goes through the liver, too. It gets big if it has too much work to do. If you drink too much, the liver can get sick. There is a disease called hepatitis, or *miskoniwâspinêw*, when the liver gets sick and some people turn yellow." I stopped speaking, and Alex tried to explain these concepts. They weren't translated as one word but as descriptive phrases.

Cree sounds so different from English. Alex's voice was deep, and the words were sort of down in his throat, more guttural, more musical. With his eyes, he was engaging with the Cree speakers in the room. A couple of times, he asked Martha, a Community Health Representative (CHR), how she would translate my words. They spoke Cree back and forth. I casually stretched out my wrist from the sleeve of my navy sweater and looked at my watch. The morning of our first day was almost over. At this rate, how would we meet the target in the grant proposal titled "Developing a Medical Vocabulary in Cree"?

Two women Elders, Dorothy and Amanda, wore coloured floral-and-white kerchiefs, mementos from times gone by, when some Russians in Moose Factory married into the community. Dorothy looked older, with a tired face. She and her friend Amanda spoke to me, Greg translating. "We both delivered babies for many years. Sometimes in the bush, out on the trapline. Sometimes in small cabins. We would usually have a wood fire to boil water, to sterilize the knife we used to cut the baby's cord and the string to tie it. The fire keeps the new mother and the baby warm. Mostly the babies were fine. Sometimes a woman would go into her birthing time early, and the baby would be small."

Greg nodded to me. Did I have questions? "So, what did you call it if the woman went into labour early? In English, we call that premature labour. And what would you do?"

Another linguistic dance flowed between Greg and the women. Then Alex stepped in with an answer in English. "We call that *wîpac âhkosiw*. We would help the baby stay warm, right on the mother's breast. We would wrap the baby in furs. We could make a small bed that did not lose the heat from a wetted, green inner tree bark lined with fur for the baby to sleep in. Sometimes, the smallest babies would die, but many did not." We now had a Cree phrase for "premature labour" and one for "newborn" — *oshki-awâshish(ak)*.

Martha, the CHR, also wanted to share. She spoke to me first in English, then in Cree to the others. "I, too, have used wetted green bark. It can be flexibly moulded, and it dries in the shape of a cast around a broken limb. I learned this from the Elders. They taught me how to make a splint to keep a broken limb straight and to protect it before I transfer the patient to Moose Factory. I'm happy the Elders are there to teach me. I didn't know about using bark to make a cast or that kind of first aid in my CHR training in Sudbury."

We had similar ideas. We had both learned how to cast a broken limb, only using different materials. I took my time, speaking slowly, which was not my custom, knowing English was not their first language. At first, I felt that I was the professional. Then I noticed how patiently the Anishinaabe were explaining things to me, the woman who spoke no Cree. My inexperience dawned on me. I had not delivered babies by the light of a wood fire or managed a broken arm in the bush, though I had worked with limited resources on Lake Temagami.

Martha looked over at me. "A lot of people get sick with coughing. Sometimes they lose weight and die. Sometimes they get better. Sometimes they need antibiotics, and sometimes they don't. Why can a cough be so many different sicknesses?" Greg and Dorothy took time to ask that question to the others in Cree. A few of them nodded. One spoke quietly, then Greg turned to me.

"The Elders know about TB. Many had this when they were younger. Coughing, losing weight, and being sent to the sanatorium. The trapper said that last year his brother also had a cough, lost weight, and died. But it was lung cancer." Now our dictionary had "cancer," *êkâ kâ-kinitokotâniwak âhkosiwin*, and "TB," *minîwâtâmêw*.

I went on to try to explain the difference between viruses (*âkosiwin manicôsh*) that did not need antibiotics and bacteria (*âhkosiwi-manicôsh*) that did, and that pneumonia (*pâhkihpanê*) was an infection in the lungs. Greg turned on a projector and showed a slide we had made of the lungs and the respiratory system, labelled in Cree. The Elders nodded and talked excitedly among themselves. They pointed at the image projected onto the wall, asking Dorothy, Greg, and Alex questions.

Perhaps I, too, could be useful here. I reached into my brown leather doctor's bag and pulled out my stethoscope. I passed it around, offering my back for the Elders to listen to my breathing. Slow, deep breaths, in and out. The Elders chuckled as they tried it, sometimes getting the stethoscope on backwards, and took turns listening to each other. They spoke to each other in Cree, those slushy, guttural sounds punctuated by slow laughs. And then, still laughing, they called out, "We're taking a smoke break to further test out our lungs!" Martha and I shared a discreet smile. This was fun. We were doing it. We were finding the right *shared* words.*

⸻

Martha was flying back up the James Bay coast to Fort Albany, and I went with her, knowing it would be a great chance to keep looking at health and life in the North through each other's eyes. We would

---

*The Cree entries in this chapter can be found in a newer medical dictionary. Since our workshop in the 1980s, there has been additional work to develop medical vocabularies in Cree, OjiCree, and Ojibwe, and the words have been updated. Greg Spence, in Fort Albany, was the team leader of the Cree vocabulary project. See *Cree Medical Dictionary: A Handbook for Health Care Providers* (Sioux Lookout, ON: Sioux Lookout Meno Ya Win Health Centre, 2011), slmhc.on.ca/assets/files/traditional-healing/medical_dictionary_cree.pdf.

continue our work up there and share what we'd done in Timmins with other Elders who might be able to help us refine the words and phrases we had created.

This was my first time in Fort Albany. We stayed in a guest house run by the priest. Martha had promised something special, a supper under the open sky, an hour's Ski-Doo drive away.

We loaded up. I wore a borrowed snowsuit, helmet, and boots. My much-loved deerskin gauntlets, embroidered with beads, came up to my elbows and still smelled of the smoke from tanning. An Elder had given them to me on a previous trip, and they made me proud — an invited guest in the home and world of another culture. I had been asked to help the Anishinaabe on their terms. I could help write the grant proposal and share medical knowledge. But the decisions about what the priorities were and why it was important to develop the Cree language to handle new concepts had been made by the Ojibwe-Cree Cultural Centre after discussion with the Elders. They were building their own history and their own resources.

The air was biting cold. We roared along on the Ski-Doo, my arms awkwardly wrapped around Martha's waist. The snow crunched beneath us. The sky above dazzled, fiercely blue bright. The air crackled. Snarling, the machine choked to a standstill as Martha cut the gas, and we shuddered to a stop.

"Here. Here is where we'll make the fire." Martha gathered twigs, branches, and bark. She scooped handfuls of low-bush cranberries into a small tin pot over the fire, cooking them till they softened to a warm sauce. Goose wrapped around two wooden sticks hissed as the fat drizzled onto the fire. Another small tin pot held tea soup — flour, tea, broth.

We sat on the Ski-Doo, relishing roast goose dipped and swirled in the cranberry sauce. The goose had been shot and dressed the night before.

As dusk set in, the last streaks of sunlight shot through the pillows of ombré clouds, violet-grey at the horizon and fading upward into light mauve-lilac. Darkness dropped, blue-black. Shivers of light flickered up, swirling shimmers of the northern lights. Martha smiled as she gazed up.

Then her radio phone crackled. "Return to the nursing station. We have an acute abdomen, fourteen-year-old girl. Right lower quadrant pain."

We donned our helmets and jumped on the Ski-Doo. Snow swirled around us as we raced the hour back to Fort Albany. We geared down to a stop and clumsily, in our bulky Ski-Doo suits, got off the vehicle and tramped into the station, stomping the snow off our boots and clothing and unfastening our helmets as we entered. Martha's colleague was there and explained the situation.

"She came in an hour ago. The pain has moved from her belly button down to the right. She has vomited once. I have taken her blood to check the white blood cell count. It wasn't too high, but it's early. It might go up. I did a pregnancy test on her urine, and it was negative, but her last period was over five weeks ago, and it was not an early morning urine specimen, so she still might be pregnant."

We looked over at Betty, a plump teenage girl who was crying and whispering to herself in Cree. She clutched her abdomen.

Martha spoke to the young woman, then nodded to me. "I've explained that we will have to fly her to the hospital. It could be appendix, or a pregnancy in her fallopian tube, or a pelvic infection."

Martha then went over to the radio phone and hailed the Moose Factory Zone Hospital. "We have an acute abdomen. Young teenage girl. The white count isn't up, and the beta HCG pregnancy test is negative, but she is vomiting and her temp is up. Might be an appendix or an ectopic pregnancy. Could be pelvic inflammatory disease."

"Roger that," crackled the response. "This is Al Hart. We'll have the O.R. ready just in case."

I asked if I could speak, and grabbed the mic. "Al Hart? Were you at St. Jo's in Hamilton?"

"That's right. Who's asking?"

"Gretchen Roedde. You taught me pediatrics. I'm working for Treaty 9 and the Cultural Centre!"

"Long time, no talk!"

We arranged to send Betty out by air ambulance and loaded the frightened girl onto a stretcher, carefully explaining in Cree what was to happen. Family gathered around for the next few hours while we waited for the plane. We were all relieved to hear the thrumming of its motor on its approach. We watched the plane land near the nursing station. "*Meegwetch*," Betty said, thanking us as the paramedics lifted her into the plane.

Martha and I stayed behind, quiet. As the medivac took off, we looked past its retreating shadow to the blaze of the northern lights, winking and swirling merrily in the vast blackness. Martha's eyes met mine. We trusted each other. We did not need to speak.

~ 7 ~

WINDIGO WELCOME

One day, after two years on Lake Temagami, I went down on my knees on the green plywood floor to pray for a change. I had been able to travel north to work on the Cree medical vocabulary. A babysitter, Sue, came in the day; Jim managed okay in the evening. When I had returned ten days later, I was able to continue breastfeeding, laying the plastic tube of an IV bag filled with dextrose and water alongside my breast so that my daughter's suckling would bring the milk back in. I could balance my life as a mother and a doctor. But, I thought, if we lived in town, I wouldn't have to haul water. I would have a lot more time.

In the spring of 1980, we went looking for homes that had running water in Haileybury, on Lake Temiskaming. We found a large one-hundred-year-old home surrounded by fruit and lilac trees that overlooked the lake. As there had been no offers in the two years it had sat unsold, we were able to buy it for twenty-six thousand dollars, and we moved in that May. Our family had a home in which we could put down new roots.

Jim's commute to Bear Island was two hours and another five if he needed to visit government archives in either Toronto or Ottawa. I could do a little local clinical work and continue working with Bear Island, helping their CHR and National Native Alcohol and Drug Abuse Program (NNADAP) worker with community health activities and seeing patients at the clinic once a month. Doreen and I would do house calls, with immunization supplies in my backpack. I could go up to Matatchewan with Lois Boston, a nurse from the Caribbean working for the Medical Services Branch, which managed First Nations health care. It was there that I saw my first moose kept as a pet, fenced in and fed through the winter to the delight of the twenty families who lived on this small reserve.

I could also take the train north to Timmins to keep working for Treaty No. 9, now called the Nishnawbe Aski Nation (NAN), and for the Ojibwe-Cree Cultural Centre. On the train home one day, I met a colleague, Brian Primrose, who remembered me from med school at McMaster. He was the medical officer of health in the region around Lake Temiskaming and was doing public health training. He was worried about some unmet needs. "This region has the highest teenage pregnancy rate in the province," he explained, "and the highest abortion rate for teenagers, and the highest rate of cancer of the cervix." In five minutes we had decided that I would start a teenage birth control clinic at the local health unit one day a week, which seemed manageable with a small baby. The next week, I found a grandmotherly neighbour, June Nabb, who agreed to babysit that one day a week.

Jim was travelling extensively, but when he was home he worked out of an office on our second floor. I did my teen clinic once a week and wondered how I would continue my plans to help train Indigenous health workers. I noticed an ad in a global public health journal for a course called "Teaching Primary Health Care," at the Liverpool School of Tropical Medicine. It was expensive — tens of thousands of pounds for three months. In the same journal, I saw a notice for a World Health Organization fellowship. I applied for both and was accepted.

As Jim had been raised in a family with a professional father and a mother who stayed home until the children were in school, he'd assumed I'd do the same. My absences for work, a few days at a time, were a growth experience for us all. I would leave bottles of formula or breast milk behind, express my milk when I was away and get breast-feeding re-established when I returned. Sometimes I could take Anna with me; First Nations people were fine having a nursing baby around.

By the time she was nine months old, Anna had decided to wean herself off breast milk; this made leaving her a little easier.

I knew how difficult this juggling act had been for Jim, so I was thrilled when he encouraged me to take the fellowship, even though this would mean leaving the family for three months. "We'll be fine. If I have a work trip, I can leave Anna with June Nabb. Or I can bring Anna down to my parents." Anna was nineteen months old at the time.

On my flight over to England, I was frightened. I had been out of school for years. I had lived in the bush, hauled water, and cared for a baby while having very limited professional experience. I wondered how I would manage away from my home. I wept every day I was away, missing my family — that hopeful little girl, that supportive husband — so badly. My African classmates had been away from their own children for longer; some were pursuing master's degrees after this three-month course. They envied me for only being away for a short time.

As it happened, two months into the course, walking on the way home to my students' residence, I was hit by a car when it ran a red light. It was a week before the fracture in my knee was diagnosed, and miraculously Jim was able to get an emergency passport, entrust our daughter to his parents' care, and fly to Liverpool for my surgery. He looked after me for a month as I convalesced and completed the course. We flew home together. Sporting a cast up to mid-thigh, and hobbling on crutches, we arrived at my in-laws' door. Anna, now twenty-two months old, looked up at me, and then turned to her grandparents, saying "Who is that lady?" My heart sank. To have been forgotten by my baby, whom I'd wept for daily — that break took longer to heal than my knee. I was grateful for a family who would care for their grand-child while I pursued my career and for a husband who supported those choices. Jim's sister's mother-in-law, Maria, came home with us to help with Anna and meals as my fracture healed. Maria was a godsend, and her culinary prowess was unparalleled. I still dream of her mocha walnut torte and the pound of butter in its icing.

The following year, the Liverpool School asked me to return as faculty. Jim thought we should have another child instead, and in September

1982, our son was born. In keeping with Scottish tradition, he was given several names, one each to honour my brother, Jim's father, and the doctor who delivered him. We called him Alec, the Scottish version of the name of our Cree friend Alex Spence. This time around, I asked my GP, Dr. McDermott, to induce me early. I was already huge. He agreed. Alec arrived on this earth weighing nine pounds, nine ounces. No epidural, six hours of labour, and a healthy mom and baby. This time, no rainstorms. And we returned to a home with running water. But a week later, Jim had to leave. The land claim trial had begun, and Jim's testimony would take several months. I got very little sleep between breastfeeding our son and coping with an irate three-year-old, who wept bitterly for her dad and was furious at a new baby. One night, I simply put Alec in his bassinet, shut the crib in the washroom downstairs, and went to an upstairs bedroom. I assume he cried in the night for food or comfort, but I had nothing to give.

I kept up with the teen clinic once a week as I could manage breastfeeding, and it was good to have colleagues with whom to socialize. I never shared my fatigue and sadness with the nurses.

One weekend I had decided to take the kids to see their dad, hoping they'd sleep on the overnight train. They did not. The rumbling noises of the train on its tracks and the lonely whistle as we came to crossings muffled the sound of my weeping.

After several months of a tough commute between Northern Ontario and Toronto, we were able to rent an apartment in Toronto for a few weeks. The lawyer for the land claim, Bruce Clark, had already rented a house for his family. Bruce was white but had lived in the far north, in Indigenous communities, as a child. His goal was to make First Nations legal history.

Chief Gary Potts, who remains a close friend, was leading the fight for acknowledgement of the community's ownership over their traditional lands. As Gary explained,

> The English Crown agents of genocide, on the payroll of
> the Ontario Crown, came to n'Dakimenan (Our Land)
> in 1901. Our people learned their habits and tried to

placate the outsiders, avoiding a major confrontation with these agents until the latter part of the 1960s. This meant ignoring harassment, such as lands and forests or ministry of natural resources employees coming into the community to confiscate legally caught game and fish. We were not allowed to hunt on our own lands, even to feed our hungry families. But when the construction of year-round roads into the centre of our homeland began, we had to fight the Ontario Crown. These "agents of genocide" came into the home of one of our community, Johnny Katt, and took his stove so he could not cook. Our legal initiative began in 1973 with a caution* registered under the Ontario Land Title Act on "Crown Land" within our Homeland to stop the Ontario Government from building a resort on Maple Mountain. Our people's name for this place is Chee-Bai-Ging (the Place Where the Spirit Goes After the Body Dies).

As the lawyer and the historian were based in Toronto for the trial, the families often visited. On those occasions, we could pool resources and hire a babysitter for all the kids. One night the four adults went out to dinner. As we worked our way through a lovely meal at a downtown Toronto restaurant, Ji and Bruce argued fact and strategy. By filing the caution, the buying and selling of property around Lake Temagami, potentially still owned by the Bear Island Band, was halted, which helped pressure the provincial government to settle the claim. Bruce's wife and I chatted about our children and the strain the land claim was putting on our families. Bruce had given up his previous supports in order to work on the land claim — wealth, a private plane, community prestige — and was

---

*A caution is a legal term that limits development, as there is a question regarding the ownership of the land.

battling a system that was decidedly unfair. He was full of idealism and had taken on the Bear Island case for the same small stipend as Jim. As the lawyer, he had to keep orchestrating the trial, a tremendous pressure.

As the trial progressed, various Elders had come down to Toronto to testify, including Kush Kush (Michael Paul), who was the last living member of the community who knew how to do the sacred shaking tent ceremony. The province's own archaeologist outlined the validity of petroglyphs on Lake Temagami and the canoe styles that showed the same band had continuously inhabited the area for several thousand years. Jim had painstakingly traced family trees back to the time of the Royal Proclamation of 1763. This document was identified as a key resource, as it stated that prior to 1763, British interests were subject to "great fraud and abuses." The Proclamation stated that any negotiations to acquire Indigenous land had to be made with representatives of the Crown, not with "settler" governments or provinces. The Bear Island land claim was being argued with just such a settler government: the Supreme Court of Ontario.

For those months of the trial, either I had to travel with two crying kids and arrive exhausted in Toronto or Jim had to make a six-hour drive to spend the weekend at home irritable and stressed. One night while I was home alone, I called Alec's godmother, Mae Katt. I told her, "Mae, I am so tired. I have enough sleeping pills to kill myself. Tell me what to do."

"Gretch, put the pills away, far away. Call me in the night if you feel bad. I will call you in the morning." She did. I told no one else, neither my doctor nor Jim, how I felt. I healed others, not myself. And how could I let our side down? The land claim was important. The courts and the provincial government were stacked against us. Jim had to be in Toronto. I had to be up north. To admit my own feelings seemed an unforgiveable sign of weakness.

Mae kept in touch, and our many ties meant she respected our family both personally and professionally. Her emotional support allowed me to survive, to parent my own children, and to keep working to carry out my dream of training First Nations health workers up north.

Frank McKay was the health program director for the Windigo Tribal Council, north of Sioux Lookout, in Nishnawbe Aski Nation. To this day, he remains the best leader for whom I have ever worked. The communities he represented wanted their own trained health workers and did not think the CHRs who'd trained at a community college farther south had the right skills. Frank explained, "Many of those trainees drop out, especially those from the far northern reserves. It's too hard to be away from family for so long and too tough to adapt to living in a 'white' environment."

I could relate, given my own time away from my family learning how to train health workers in Third World settings. This had included writing curriculum. Frank wanted local input to what the health workers would be trained to do. I figured we could talk to the communities and find out their priorities, then Frank would guide me to write the curriculum and format skills training sessions. We'd need Indigenous trainers. We could do the training up north under actual job conditions.

I flew up to Sioux Lookout. It's actually a long way to go from where I live, at the eastern border of Ontario near Quebec, to the western boundary with Manitoba. It's an hour-and-a-half drive to North Bay, a one-hour flight to Sudbury, then on to Sault St. Marie, Thunder Bay, and Sioux. This trip takes a couple of days, as you have to break the trip in Thunder Bay.

When I got into Sioux, I met Frank at the tribal council office. He said, "We're going to need money. I can organize the communities. Your job is to manage the white world. Help us get the money, write the proposal, find trainers, write the reports. That way you bring skills from the white world when you come to the Chiefs' meetings, and you write up the notes based on the spoken words from the Elders. We can do this if we all work together."

Once I was home, I figured that I'd need to learn some new skills — and quickly. I called up Vic Neufeld and Peter Tugwell, at McMaster. These two teachers from my medical school have remained mentors my whole life.

"How do I get money for a health worker training program up north?" I asked Vic.

"Come on down, visit your in-laws in Ancaster, and spend a few days with us. We'll get some ideas together."

I took his advice, and when I arrived, Vic and Peter gave me a book of foundations to look through. Peter suggested that I get a National Health Grant to do a feasibility study while looking for larger sources of funds. Three looked promising: a medical charity run by physicians (PSI); Roncalli, a Roman Catholic foundation; and the Donner Foundation. After two days I had proposals for all three, as well as one for a National Health Grant.

Within a few months, I had heard back from all the agencies, and we had been awarded grants from all of them. We were rolling.

For the next trip up to the Sioux, we hired three trainers, Mae, Nellie, and Liz.

My friend Mae Katt, the nurse from Bear Island, had been working at the Zone Hospital.

Nellie Beardy had been a CHR, had her grade seven, and spoke OjiCree. Her husband, Stan, was a Chief, and she was from Windigo Tribal Council, so she had a perspective on how the CHRs could be better trained to suit the real job situation.

Liz Roberts was a physician who had been working at the Sioux Lookout Zone Hospital for years. Liz was ready to leave the colonial hospital run by white people, to work directly on behalf of First Nations.

Frank arranged for us to meet at the tribal council office with the Elders and other community leaders who had flown into Sioux Lookout to plan the project.

The community health leaders gave valuable input to the task of drafting some ideas for the training. There was a big desire for mother and child care and obstetrics. People needed to know how to deliver babies, and they wanted to learn how to suture. People often got sick, so they needed to know about infections and how to do first aid on the trapline. Whatever we taught the health workers, the communities wanted to learn as well.

I took the notes home and churned out curriculum, learning objectives based on these themes, rocking my infant son as I wrote. The plan was to do the training in a modular format: a mother and child health

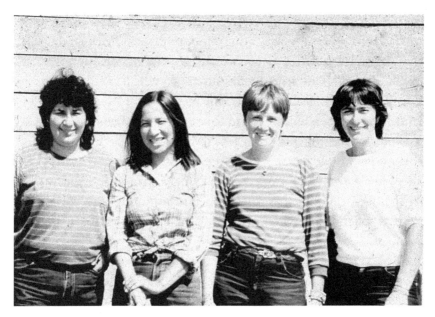

Left to right: Mae Katt, Nellie Beardy, Gretchen Roedde, and Liz Roberts, Windigo Paramedic Training Team.

module for a few weeks in Muskrat Dam; then infections in another module in Sachigo Lake. The communities would be responsible for billeting the trainees and trainers and arranging a training space. Everyone was welcome, and anyone who had skills could join as a welcome resource. We had done something similar at Bear Island when my brother Steve, an E.R. doc, came to teach a first aid course, and Vicki's dad, Maurice, who'd been a paramedic in the war, volunteered to help teach suturing.

Though I'd left the kids at home with their dad, I brought a voice recording of Alec. He participated in our OB training: the sound of my own crying baby to add some realism!

~

We were in the old band office in Muskrat Dam; kids and adults alike crowded around, looking in the windows. A couple of brave souls had ventured in to where we were teaching the CHR trainees. Actually, we had renamed the workers the Windigo Paramedic Program trainees. An arrangement had been made with Confederation College, in Thunder Bay, to accredit the program, which would be run by the Windigo Tribal Council. If this was successful here, in an area with strong leadership, we could expand to other tribal councils. We intended to use role play to teach, to help make the learning enjoyable, and to build on the Indigenous sense of fun and teasing. We were thrilled when an external team of evaluators who had worked in Third World as well as First Nations communities gave us a very positive assessment, which we were able to present to our funding agencies.

Mae was playing *kokum*, or grandmother, dressed with an old kerchief and padding under her clothes. Everyone was laughing. She was

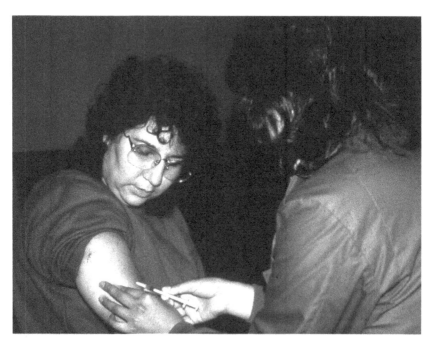

Mae Katt and Nellie Beardy teaching about injections.

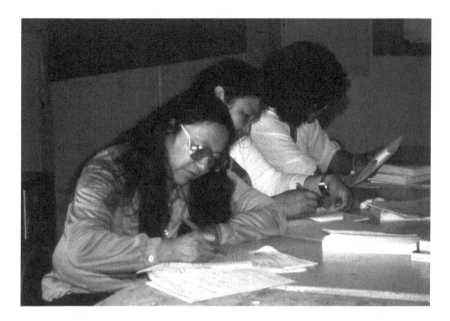

Trainees writing exams.

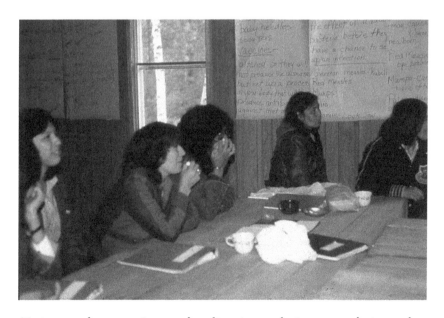

Trainees and community members listening to the instructor during a class.

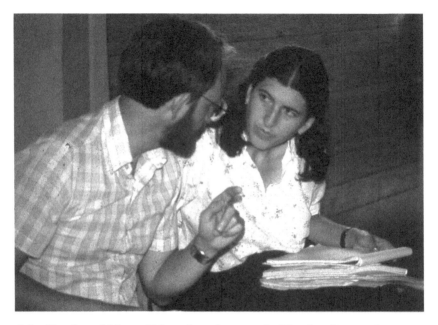

John Frank and Nancy Edwards evaluating the Windigo Paramedic Program.

going to show how to deliver a baby. Nellie was playing her pregnant daughter, who was giving birth in the community as the weather was bad and she could not get out to the Zone Hospital in Sioux.

Nellie lay down, pulled a blanket over herself, and made convincing labouring cries. We had a rubber ring to represent the birth canal and a baby doll. *Kokum* was busy getting ready to deliver the baby, muttering to herself in OjiCree. Kids giggled at the windows; the students were laughing, too, as were Nellie and Mae. Liz encouraged our "labouring" mother. "Now push! I know it hurts. Just take a deep breath and PUSH hard with each pain. Then pant in between. Then push again." Then Alec's first performance before an audience was upon us. I hit play when the baby doll was duly delivered. Alec's wail filled the room as he cried for his mom, as hungry as he would be when I returned to be a mother, instead of a doctor and teacher.

At night, resting in my billeted room, I gradually fell asleep while listening to drumming and singing from a traditional music group practising outside for an upcoming celebration. "Ahee!" rang out the chanting sounds, and the footsteps from the dancers pounded gently on the ground. I felt like I was in a universal womb, cocooned with the soothing sound of a Great Mother's heartbeat around me.

∽ 8 ∾

PORCUPINE HIDING

I continued my work as a teacher when, after initially postponing the job, I joined the faculty at Liverpool School of Tropical Medicine to teach Third World students every spring for three years (1983–85). I would go to England and teach that same course, "Teaching Primary Health Care," I had taken when my first child was small. This time, late spring 1983, the family came, too. After a sleepless flight to Manchester, an hour's journey on the wrong (left) side of the road, Jim drove our foursome up to the house that would be our temporary home. Our new landlord, Eddy, greeted us warmly as we arrived. The top floor was our flat, he explained. He invited us into his home.

"You guys must be shattered!" he said. "Sorry, the flat is not quite ready. Let's make you all some tea, and we have juice for the kiddos. This is Syl. She runs the house, and our family's life!" Syl bustled in with cups and saucers and immediately reached for Anna's hand. "Come with me, luv. You'll give us a hand in the kitchen, all right?"

Anna, then five, instantly forgot any fatigue and allowed herself to be led into the kitchen. None of us knew that a decades-long friendship would spring from this moment. Syl pointed out some black-and-white portraits on the wall. "Those are our four — Dionne, Sara, Michaela, and Marlene. They're in school just now, but you'll meet them later." By the time Jim and I had finished our tea and the kids their juice, the flat was ready. Anna had found a renewed energy after the sleepless night

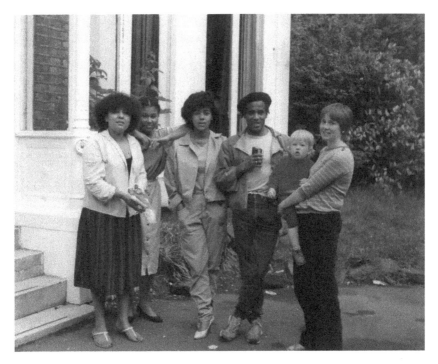

With Eddy and Sylvia Amoo, Liverpool, 1984.

and bounded up the stairs. Both Syl and the secretary from the school had found some toys for us, and soon Alec was playing with them while Jim and I unpacked. The next day, the nanny we'd hired, Cassie, a relative of friends back home, arrived, ready to take the kids to Sefton Park to see the ducks. Cassie was marvellous with the kids, who were delighted by her thick Yorkshire accent.

We settled in well, Jim doing most of the cooking after driving me to work in the mornings, though it was my job to get up with Alec in the night. We all had our own rooms in the flat.

A short while later, I discovered I was pregnant. I wasn't worried, as I had done my own pre-natal care for several months when we were living on Lake Temagami. I figured I could manage that until we got home, given that as a non-national I wasn't sure how I would get a doctor.

I loved my students, who had come from countries like Bhutan, a Buddhist kingdom in the Himalayas, and Papua New Guinea, on the other side of the earth. Many were from countries in Africa and wore long, flowing robes and turbans. All religions were represented.

One day we lecturers took our thirty students on a bus tour of Liverpool, where they took in various Beatles haunts, as well as areas with subsidized housing. The students were surprised. These seedy tenements, examples of lapses in housing standards, seemed luxurious to them. "Please, Doctor, serious, these are given to people to live in by the government? This is a lucky country. But why are those old people walking alone in the street? Where are their children? Don't the children take care of the Elders here?" The students were shocked to visit a nursing home. "Why are these people living here? Why have their children not taken them in? Maybe this country is not so lucky after all. Families don't look after each other here."

During my time there, one of my colleagues suffered two losses in a short space of time when his aunt and his mother died within days of each other. He continued to work, British stiff upper lip and all. When the students learned of his bereavement from the school secretary, they asked me what they should do, in this culture, to share his sadness. "In Africa, we would give him money for the funeral feast." I asked the school secretary what was customary here in England. "We just let him have his privacy," she said. "He wouldn't want anyone to make a fuss."

Many of the students did maternal health care in their own countries. They would eagerly ask how my pregnancy was progressing. "Soon you will be big with the baby! We are so happy for you."

The school term was coming to a close, and we were set to visit family friends elsewhere in England before returning to Canada. But as we headed out to the loaded car, I started to bleed. I explained to Jim what was happening, made my way back into the house, and slowly and carefully walked up the flights of stairs to the third-floor flat. Jim and the kids followed. Syl had seen us get ready to depart, only to come back into the house, and she came upstairs herself. "What's wrong?"

I told her that I was bleeding and would rest for a few hours, hoping it would stop.

She was insistent. "I'm getting my GP here straight away," she said.

An hour later, a kindly doctor arrived with his medical bag. "I'm just going to see how things are." He felt my abdomen and listened for the baby's heartbeat. "I'm going to give you some progesterone, a hormone to try to keep the baby. You just rest in bed. No travelling for now. I will see you again tomorrow."

Jim called our friends to cancel.

True to his word, the doctor came daily, but the bleeding did not stop. "You'd best go 'round to the Women's Hospital. You need to see the consultant there. You'll need to be admitted."

Jim drove us over to the Liverpool Women's and Children's Hospital, where I was tucked into bed by caring nurses. The obstetrician came in to examine me. "I think we need you to get a scan," he said. We don't have a machine here, cutbacks you know. You'll need to go over to another hospital." So the nurses got me dressed again and into a waiting black taxicab, and off I went.

Once at the newer modern hospital, I was taken up to the radiology suite and into a room for an ultrasound. As I watched the screen, I saw the fetus detach from the womb. "No fetal heart," said the technician. "It looks like the baby has died. We'll get you back to the Women's as you may need some help if the miscarriage isn't complete." Tight-lipped, I allowed myself to be taken back in another taxi to my waiting hospital bed.

The consultant called Jim, and when he arrived, explained that our baby had died. "Fetal demise. You're in your second trimester, so I think we will need to do a dilatation and curettage under an anaesthetic to empty the womb surgically, to make sure there is no tissue left inside that can cause bleeding."

As the senior registrar, or Chief Resident, wheeled me down to the operating room, he said, "You're a doctor. Don't take this too hard. You know that one in five pregnancies ends in miscarriage."

This callous remark exacerbated my pain. I was stunned. I was barely holding it together.

Jim stayed outside the O.R., which was just as well, because the anaesthetist came over to say that as I was Rh-negative I would need Rhogam to prevent complications in future pregnancies. "No need! My husband is also Rh-negative," I told him. "Ah," said the doctor, "but what if he is not the baby's father?" I was angry, and sad, and empty, and said nothing. But I refused the Rhogam.

When it was all over and we were back in the flat, I took to my bed and did not come out. I would see no one. No students. No colleagues. My daughter told me much later that she peeked under the door to see if I really was inside. Syl took Anna under her wing, bringing Anna on her trips around Liverpool to check on the other flats the family managed. Eddy would come up, concern marking his face, on my infrequent forays out of the room, and Syl would bring me sweet-smelling freesias. Those golden blooms can still bring on an overwhelming sense of loss.

But Syl was the only one who could break through my prickly porcupine exterior. Jim couldn't reach me, and I felt numb around the still-chattering children. I hid myself inside my room, barely able to read my usual fare of mindless murder mysteries. We packed up our belongings and made the great transition back to Manchester, then to Toronto, then home to Northern Ontario.

I carried on with my own heartbreak, that secret sorrow. No one had known I was pregnant before we left, so back in Canada I could almost pretend nothing had happened except my teaching. I, too, could hide my anguish with a stiff upper lip.

~ 9 ~

COYOTE TRICKSTER

Our time in Liverpool, though filled with loss, had been an important break from the political struggles we had faced at home, in Northern Ontario. The Teme-Augama Anishnabai, or Deep Water People, did not win their Supreme Court case. Bruce Clark did not take the loss well. This was also an enormous blow to Jim, as so much of his work seemed wasted. Judge Steele had made negative comments about everyone who had testified on Temagami's behalf. Chief Gary Potts, who had led his community to fight for their land, remained strong and determined. Vicki had an interesting perspective. "The trouble with the land claim is that Gary Potts wants to be the lawyer and Bruce Clark wants to be the Indian chief. Jim is the only one who knows what his role is."

The appeals process began, but the band wanted to use a Toronto firm. Interpreting this as a demotion and refusing to stay on in an official capacity, Bruce packed up his family and moved away. While the legal machinery ground along through the 1980s, protests representing the different interest groups were a regular occurrence, usually on the Red Squirrel Road outside of Temagami. Loggers wanted the caution lifted so development could continue. Environmentalists wanted to preserve the last remaining stand of old-growth red pine in North America. First Nations activists wanted recognition for the un-ceded title. Group after group protested in the 1980s. In late 1989, protesters who came to support Bear Island included Frank Beardy, of Big Trout Lake, who I had worked with up north, and Elders from Big Trout Lake and Muskrat Dam.

But still there was no settlement. After Bruce was excluded from the land claim appeal, he teamed up with a few disaffected individuals, mostly angry young men. Bruce had convinced them that previously unused legal and historical documents, like a 1704 British Privy Council judgment, could still support their claim.

Meanwhile, Jim had begun working with all opposing groups, environmentalists, and loggers, Indigenous and not, as the chair of the Wendabun Stewardship Authority, which advised the Ontario provincial government on how the stand of old growth red pines should be used. He'd also contributed to a Sierra Club book on Indigenous Peoples and forests and how to harmonize opposing perspectives. This book came with me later on one of my global health assignments, as a gift to an environmentalist colleague in Bhutan, which, to this day, is the only carbon neutral country in the world and which respects the rights of traditional peoples living in forest regions.

⁓

In 1993, Bruce led a dozen angry men to our home to conduct a citizen's arrest of Jim, claiming wrongly that he was hiding documents related to the 1704 Privy Council decision. An Ontario Provincial Police (OPP) officer, Dana Mclean, whom I'd known since our children were small, escorted me to each of the men surrounding our home, all of whom had been patients, to give them each a notice of trespass and tearfully ask that they leave. I didn't understand how it could all go so wrong. Later, when I had to testify at a trial over the events of that day, I broke down on the stand. "For twenty years we've been working with First Nations people. I just don't understand how we became the enemy." My sobs echoed through the courtroom, and a worried murmuring could be heard by the others in the room — people from Bear Island, court reporters, cops, lawyers.

The judge looked over at me. "There will be a short recess while Dr. Roedde composes herself."

The price of admission to a complex world.

———

In 2016, as part of a series of regional perspectives to reflect on the Truth and Reconciliation Commission, a workshop was held in Temagami, facilitated by Dick and Vicki Grant. The fact that few history classes are taught about the Royal Proclamation of 1763 or the 1704 Privy Council judgment* and what they meant for the First Nations whose lands have been misappropriated was raised by Dick Grant as an error that needs to be corrected for true integration to occur. The work of the Wendabun Stewardship Authority and Jim's work with the band were cited as positive examples of integration.

Wayne Potts, on leave as vice-principal of Attawapiskat First Nation, spoke eloquently of the damage in that community, the suicides, the misused money from the mine on the reserve. Robin Potts, niece to both Gary and Wayne, spoke movingly of how the white canoe camps had raised money to help bring back the traditional style of canoe building. Kids from Bear Island, on scholarships to the camp, were building these birchbark canoes alongside white kids.

I wept through the afternoon. Our family had sacrificed money, physical comfort, and personal safety living in a harsh environment, as well as time together as a family, but had gained so much in bearing witness to important changes. At the end of the workshop, Wayne came up to me, remembering the time I took out his cat's stitches and the time I looked after his dad at Laura McKenzie's funeral. Robin Potts also

---

*The British Privy Council judgment ruled that British colonial courts were biased against Indigenous Peoples in land claim cases and that land expropriations needed to be decided on by a specially convened constitutional court. However, this court was never formed and the ruling was forgotten.

came up to me and asked if I remembered having her to our home in Haileybury. "I was at school, getting my degree. We ran into you, and you invited us for dinner."

These are the important stories. The rest are simply footnotes.

I am reminded of the Coyote. In Indigenous teachings, the Coyote impersonated the Creator. "Old Man Coyote took up a handful of mud and out of it made people." The Coyote does make things happen. He tricks and changes and brings transformation through crazy wisdom.

A couple of years later, I had a different kind of run-in with Bear Island.

I used to do a monthly clinic at Bear Island at the band's request after we had moved to town. Having lived and worked there for two years (with Doreen Potts, whom I trained, carrying medical supplies in a backpack) back in 1978–80, and having worked with the band over the years to develop a drug and alcohol program after I moved to Haileybury, it was great to reconnect with the community.

There was now a large and well-equipped medical centre, named after Doreen Potts, where I would see patients. Doctors in busy practices are used to being given prescriptions by various medical office staff — nurses, secretaries — to sign. The doctor is usually briefed about these prescriptions — say, in the case of a narcotic order, "Yeah, she has been on this for years and never fills the script early," or whatever. For example, in my work covering for another doctor in the town of Temagami, on one day I signed about ten prescriptions from the nurse practitioner for patients I had not seen, based on her guidance. The busy medical practices I cover are too swamped for me to see every patient that I sign prescriptions for.

So at Bear Island, the Doreen Potts Health Centre was run by the community. The clinic administrator gave me some prescriptions to sign. How hard could this be? An exercise bicycle, an arm exercise machine for someone with an amputated leg. These were for vets, Indigenous persons, both men and women, who had served in the Armed Forces. Department of Veterans' Affairs (DVA) was going to pay for five pieces of exercise equipment in total. I had previously met the doctor at DVA in Kirkland Lake, and she had told me the DVA was very keen on partnerships with community. There were precedents for prescribing items such as exercise equipment for vets, equipment that would be shared with the community — in this case, Bear Island wanted an Elders' exercise program that non-vets could also access.

The clinic administrator had talked with the DVA and said it was a go. Here were the scripts to sign. I assumed someone had spoken to those vets. I signed the prescriptions and happily went off to Bangladesh for a month.

Four weeks later I came back and was sorting through my mail. There was an envelope with the return address from the chief of staff of my local hospital. The letter, copied to me, contained his response to the DVA, which was considering charging me with medical fraud. My colleague explained that I had never been involved in any similar activities, and he was vouching for my good character. I wrote letters of apology to these various fine people on Bear Island, those vets whose names had been misused without their permission. As well, I decided that since the community had just recruited a First Nations band member as a nurse, there was no longer a need for me to keep on with the monthly clinics. My friend Linda Joe Mattias (who was then the CHR) was disappointed that I was stopping the clinics, but we continued with other community health programs such as drug and alcohol training. The DVA decided, after a firm reprimand, that I was not a serious risk to the integrity of their agency.

Potential catastrophe over exercise bicycles averted.

~ 10 ~

SAGE LESSONS

As Jim and I each navigated complex work responsibilities, we became increasingly divided. As I juggled my local general practice of largely non-Indigenous patients, First Nations health projects, and short-term global health assignments in the developing world, Jim was travelling extensively throughout North America on various land claims. It was exhausting. In one three-week period I had evaluated a mother and child health project in Mali, then had flown up to Big Trout Lake in Sioux Lookout Zone to train First Nations drug and alcohol workers, and had then returned to Haileybury/New Liskeard to do a family planning clinic for adolescents. We alternated our schedules so that someone was always home with the two kids, both of them thriving in the local French Catholic school. We also helped each with our difficult vocations. Just as I had supported Jim when Bruce attacked our home, Jim had driven me through a terrible ice storm that closed highways and shut off electricity for weeks in eastern Ontario and Quebec so that I could attend a meeting in Hull about a Canadian health project in Bangladesh.

Both Jim and I had demanding vocations. We were burning ourselves and each other out. On the home front, we maintained the illusion that all was well. The whole family would attend midnight Mass at Christmas, even when our travels had kept us separated for weeks. We would often have friends over for great food and live music: I would cook up loads of food, and Jim would assemble various acoustic keyboard players and guitar players to accompany his Dobro playing long into the night, while a collective group of kids, including our own, played along on instruments or sang along with their mothers.

Not only were our professional workloads intense, but also our philosophies to our work were different. For Jim, it was the process, not the outcome, he worked for. I would get distressed that too little was changing for too much work. I am still deeply wounded that after years of sacrifice and years of family poverty, there has yet to be a settlement to the Bear Island land claim. In autumn 2014, there was yet another protest on the Red Squirrel Road near Bear Island over the unresolved Teme-Augama Anishnabai land claim.

But our work also enriched our family's lives. When our kids were small, Jim worked at an archaeological dig on Manitoulin Island, and it was amazing to watch the team sift through hundreds of years of soil to find Indigenous burial sites (dogs buried ceremoniously), beads, or coins used in trade. This experience sparked a yearly tradition, spending late August in a cabin at Providence Bay. Here we could listen to the wind in the trees and the soft lapping of the water on the shore of Lake Huron, play board games and charades with our friends John and Cathleen and daughter Alix, who had the neighbouring cottage, and watch the costumed dramas the kids would put on for the grownups. They often imitated us, far too convincingly. They usually characterized Jim and me as sitting at computers, working and looking tired.

And we were tired. I remember one time Jim had been up all night at Dick Grant's law practice, now in New Liskeard, getting some legal document or another ready for a filing deadline. Anxious and angry (*When is he coming home? He promised he would be here by midnight!*), I had paced the floor till the wee hours before finally going to bed.

Jim arrived home at eight in the morning, after having worked all night. He began loading up the car for our annual pilgrimage to Manitoulin.

As Jim packed, I got breakfast ready for us all: pancakes and bacon with loads of coffee for Jim and me. Somehow we managed to make it to Providence Bay after the usual five-hour drive, listening to CBC radio — *Quirks and Quarks* or the *Royal Canadian Air Farce* — or Dire Straits's "Sultans of Swing" and David Lindley's version of "Werewolves of London" on tapes. Though exhausted, Jim then helped with the bonfire down by the beach, and in the morning, after a run, he had *pain au chocolat* ready for the two families.

Having only one job was easy. There had been safety and power in wearing a stethoscope. When I was an intern at St. Joseph's Hospital in Toronto, in 1978, I could throw my burgundy-coloured stethoscope casually around my shoulders and walk the one block to the hospital from my home as a super woman. I could work for thirty-two hours at a stretch with no sleep. I could run from one life-threatening emergency to another, making crucial/life-saving/momentous decisions. I could manage the acute pulmonary edema with morphine and Lasix on one floor and then sprint to another patient's bedside to quickly order an ECG that showed dangerously high levels of potassium. After diagnosing the patient's failed kidney dialysis, I could prescribe the right cocktail of drugs and nutrients to bring down the potassium levels, then get the nephrologist there at two in the morning, ready to assist with putting in a new dialysis shunt because the patient's line had blocked. Cardiac arrests ("Doctor 55" was the code on the loudspeaker) were handled quickly and easily. I would arrive home exhausted, throw off my stethoscope, fall into a slumped, panicked pool of terror, and wonder how I had gotten through it all.

Not only does the stethoscope confer magical powers, but it also makes sure that all the bad things happen to the person who sits across from the one adorned with the stethoscope. I am the doctor: therefore, my kids don't get sick, my marriage won't fall apart, and I will remain illness-free.

This is a fantasy world, and I have lived there. But I also must live, like everyone else, in the world as it is.

In the year 2000, after a quarter century of marriage, we slowly ground to a halt as a family. Chief Gary Potts came up to our home in Haileybury. He asked if he could take us out on our boat on Lake

Temiskaming. It was August, a brilliant blue–sky day with a bright sun and just a few geese starting to assemble overhead, flying in their V-formation, while some started to collect and paddle in a few inlets near the marina as we took out the boat. Two pairs of loons called to each other and then ducked down under the water as they heard our motorboat approach. I was reminded of travelling with Gary on Lake Temagami as he took us to our first home on the lake. He, too, had watched his marriage to Doreen end. He, too, had struggled with the sense of loss, as Doreen had died after the divorce and her family had only reluctantly allowed him to the hospital as she lay dying over several days.

The air was cool with a light wind, but the sun warmed our faces. The water sparkled and flashed. My lower lip was trembling. I could not look at Jim. Gary could look at us both, and he held us with his gaze. His dark eyes looked at us each in turn. He puffed quietly on a pipe as he drove us around the lake, calmly guiding the tiller. He pointed up to a local landmark, Devil's Rock, a jagged rock wall facing the water and extending high up to an escarpment lined with trees. Gary explained its real name should have been translated as Spirit Rock. Early Christian whites had translated it wrong, as only Christian motifs could merit the term *spirit*, so instead it became Devil's Rock. He advised us to try to keep a sense of our own strength, to not feel broken as individuals just because the marriage had broken. "You have both served our communities. We know how much you've given. Jim, Gretchen, you have journeyed with us, on the inside of our community. You are both still with us. And we are still with you, even if you're now going to be apart." I turned my head; I did not want anyone to see my tears.

As we drove around the lake, I realized that juggling these roles of mother and wife and doctor and teacher had taken from me everything I had, but they had also made me become more than I could have imagined.

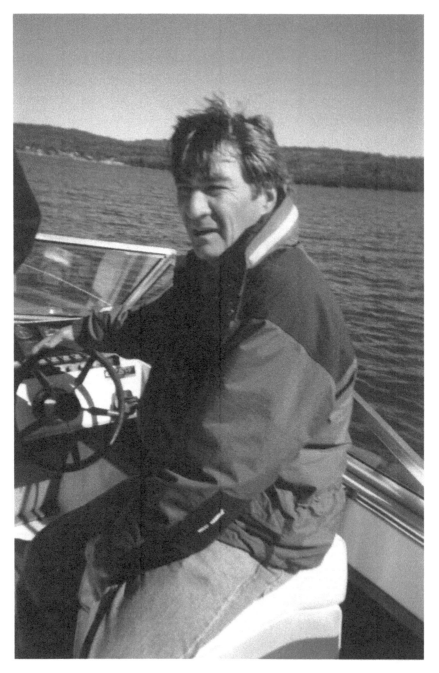

Gary Potts, driving Gretchen and Jim around Lake Temiskaming, 2000.

SECTION THREE

SHA'NGABI'HANONG / shahn-guh-bee-han-noong / Spirit Keeper of the West

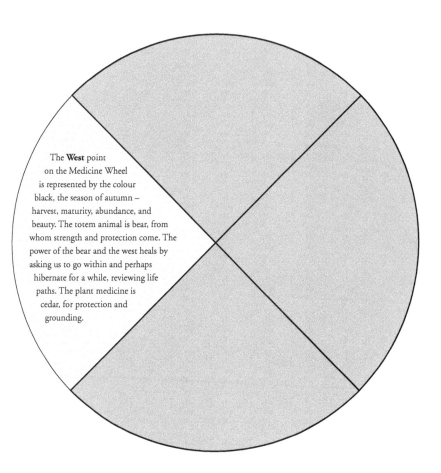

The **West** point on the Medicine Wheel is represented by the colour black, the season of autumn – harvest, maturity, abundance, and beauty. The totem animal is bear, from whom strength and protection come. The power of the bear and the west heals by asking us to go within and perhaps hibernate for a while, reviewing life paths. The plant medicine is cedar, for protection and grounding.

~ 11 ~

MAKWA (BEAR) GOES WITHIN

Fall is a complex season in the North. Some days can be cold and rainy, while others are filled to bursting with apples ripe in the trees and plums a lush yellow-orange as brilliant, warm days last late into the night. It's always a struggle to keep up with the fruit; each day I collect the apple windfalls and pick enough plums to feed the constant pot of chutney simmering on the stove. The smell of ginger and curry spices mix with the sour of some vinegar, added to offset the sweet fruit. The mix changes with each batch, always with some onions from the Mennonites at the Saturday farmer's market, but the spices change with my mood, and the apple and plum ratios depend on what's in the garden. Sometimes there are so many apples that I have to slice up a few to mix with cinnamon, nutmeg, and brown sugar and freeze in pie plates, all ready to be turned into a pie or apple crisp come winter. I remember living on Lake Temagami and the early days in my current home on Lake Temiskaming, how Jim and I would cut the apples into slices and hang them on wool strings around the house, drying and filling our home with the sweet apple scent. We would pack the dried slices into jars to keep that sweet goodness through the winter too.

Late one evening, still with the sweet spicy smell from the cooling chutney, I had a call from a nearby hospital. "Your son has been in an accident. He was thrown out of a truck and is being admitted overnight. You can pick him up in the morning."

Alec had been staying with me after living out West for a couple of years. His sister now lived in a house she owned around the corner from me and worked for one of my colleagues.

Around eight the next morning, I drove up to Englehart, thirty minutes north, and picked up my son. He seemed drowsy. The doctor on call told me to keep an eye on him. Alec was one of two kids who had been in the back of a pickup truck when the tailgate catch had loosened on the cab door, and they had both been thrown out. The other kid wasn't doing too well. The docs were waiting on an MRI (magnetic resonance imaging) in Timmins to see the extent of his head injury. I brought Alec home and put him to bed. "I'll be home in an hour or so. I just have to assist in a case in the operating room. I won't be long." I left, worried.

In the O.R., in my greens, I told my colleagues what had happened. "He seems drowsy. A bit nauseated. The docs thought he was okay to be discharged, but I'm worried his head injury may be more serious."

Pat, the other assistant in the O.R., agreed. "Go ahead, scrub out. Go home, get your son, and bring him to emerg."

This was easier said than done. Alec was indeed drowsy but had no interest in getting out of bed and into a car. I called a friend of his up the road who had been in the truck as well and had organized the first aid scene while waiting for the paramedics, his knowledge based on his ski patrol training. "Hey, Dean, I need you to help me get Alec into the car." A couple of minutes later, Dean arrived. He talked patiently to Alec.

"Okay, buddy, come on. Down the stairs, that's it. Now into the driveway, that's it. Into the car. You're okay to drive him, Gretch?"

"Sure thing." I sped off to the hospital and helped get Alec into the emergency department, where his family doctor was on call. Glen took a quick look at him, looked into his ear, and saw there was some drainage. "I think he has a skull fracture. Are you okay to take him to Timmins? They can do an MRI as soon as you get him there. It'll be quicker than waiting for an ambulance. But make sure you talk to the radiologist. We've just had word that the other kid who was with Alec had to go to

Sudbury as he was bleeding in the brain, and the radiologists missed it on his MRI."

Alec had the wristband on that they had put on him in emerg. It is usually a three-hour drive to Timmins. From time to time, Alec would look up at me drowsily. "What's with the lead foot, Mom?" I tried to joke away my own worries (about him possibly bleeding into his brain, which I was certainly not going to share), reminding Alec about my normal tendency to speed. Two-and-a-half hours later, we rolled into the Timmins Hospital parking lot and soon were in the MRI suite. I introduced myself to the radiologist. "I'm Alec's mother. I'm also a physician. I want to look at the films with you."

There was a fracture in the back of Alec's head and a subdural haematoma, or bleeding in the brain, by the fracture, as well as a *contrecoup* injury, where the front of his brain was bruised from the force of the blow at the back pushing his brain against the skull. Together with the radiologist, I called Alec's doctor at Temiskaming Hospital. The radiologist told Alec's doctor, "It's okay to manage him medically. He won't need surgery." He then told me, "Just drive him back to Temiskaming Hospital. You don't need to drive him to Sudbury for neurosurgery."

We drove the speed limit home, and Alec spent a few days in hospital until he was well enough to come home. He had lost his sense of smell and had some difficulty concentrating. In the evenings, we'd sit in the garage, Alec playing guitar and smoking a cigarette while I worked on a mosaic tile table. Normally I am unable to be still. But keeping Alec company was what I needed to do. I felt myself slowing down or, at least, trying to.

But my fast-paced life was calling. I had a quick trip to Uganda planned — just over a week, on behalf of the Irish government, to look at a training program for rural health workers. But who would look after Alec? He still needed supervision. Anna was unsure she could manage alone, and her dad could only come for a day. So Anna, ever resourceful, enlisted the help of a family friend, the doctor she worked for. Mark, who often resembles a teenager trapped in a six-foot-five body, is also a great musician. He arranged to visit Alec and jam with him. He invited

Alec over to his home around the corner and recorded him in his studio. So, while I was travelling by Jeep with a team of doctors in Uganda from village to health centre to hospital, my own home front was being cared for by family and friends. I returned home exhausted and decided it was time to schedule a long overdue screening of my own health.

My mother's mother had suffered with breast cancer, shortly after my mother, the eighth and last child, was born. My grandmother went off for treatments, leaving my mother to be cared for by sisters and a locally hired nanny. That babysitter then died in childbirth, leaving my mother with many early losses. I understood all of that later. For now, at the age of fifty-two, it was time to get a mammogram for myself. It had been five years since my previous test, longer than recommended for a woman with a family history of breast cancer. I had put it off, thinking that with my luck, it would show cancer, and I did not have time for cancer.

The mammogram did not care about my schedule. A very suspicious mass was detected in the left breast. The radiologist suggested extra views and an ultrasound. I knew what these would confirm. "Spiculated, irregular, coarse calcifications" — these were already a doctor's code words for breast cancer. Tom, my family doctor, who had delivered my son, called me to his office to tell me. It was a Monday at four thirty in the afternoon. I knew the two local surgeons would still be in their offices. "Okay, Tom, wish me luck. I'm going to try to get on the O.R. list for tomorrow."

I raced up to the hospital, definitely speeding, and ran down the corridor to Ray Rahn's office. Jake, the other surgeon, had just left. "Ray, I need your help." I handed over the mammogram print with the special views and ultrasound reports. "I know tomorrow is Tuesday, that it is Jake's O.R. day. Do you think you could both operate? Is there time to call radiology down in North Bay? We'll need them for the wire placement into the suspicious mass and to confirm you get it all with the post-op mammo through the specimen."

Ray was sure he could get it organized, and he examined me. "I don't feel anything. That's good. If it's not palpable, it's small, early, curable."

I was relieved, not only that this would be a favourable prognosis, but also that I hadn't missed something on my own breast exams. *What kind of credibility would that give for the well woman clinics I had been running in the local hospital?* I had started these in 1990, after handing over the teenage clinic to another female physician.

It was September. I dressed carefully in the morning: a warm dark-nut-brown sweater and darker brown jeans for fall; hot pink earrings and a pink necklace for breast cancer. I changed into a patient gown and wrap in the pre-op room, and then my friend Jake, the other surgeon, came to visit me, sitting on my bed. He was then seventy years old. "Gretchen, we've just had a marvellous trip to New York, to celebrate my birthday." He spoke slowly, in his English accent. "Now, don't be worried. Ray and I will both do the surgery." Then the anaesthetist, my colleague and Alec's GP, came over to explain how he would put me to sleep. Cindy, my friend and one of the nurses, wheeled me into the O.R. Surrounded by friends and colleagues, all in their greens, I drifted off to a worried, drugged unconscious state.

I woke up later, groggy. Anna came to pick me up and drove us home, ten minutes away. My daughter was now my caregiver. I slowly made my way into my house. I had binding dressings over my bleeding cut-open breast. I ignored the pain. Smiling cheerfully, I tried to put on a brave front for my children. I said little to Alec, who was still recovering. I got a new outfit ready for work the next day. I had no sick leave. I chose a pale blue lacy sweater over a tight undershirt with blue jean leggings. Somewhat stiffly, I prepared for bed, grateful for pain meds and sleeping tablets. I smiled a goodnight to Alec and waved goodbye to Anna, who had prepared our supper before going up to her own home. "I'm driving you to work tomorrow, Mum. See you in the morning!" Leaving my clothes on a hanger, I climbed into bed and slept awkwardly, painfully, waking through the night.

Morning came earlier than I expected. I was not ready to pretend to be well while being a post-operative patient. Anna picked me up, casting a worried look at the frown lines on my forehead, indicating the pain I was in. We drove together to the clinic, where we both worked. As I saw each patient, I knew that I was really not ready to be there. Angrily, I refused two requests for sick notes, for one person who had a cold and for another who had acne. It is also entirely possible, though I was on so many painkillers I cannot really remember, that I pulled up my sweater to show the blood seeping through my wound dressings to one woman and said, "I'm working. Why do you think you're too sick?"

On Monday I had received X-ray confirmation of highly probable breast cancer. Surgery had been the following day. On Wednesday and Thursday I had worked in my clinic in Haileybury. On Friday, while working at another clinic, I took a break from my work so that a nurse could change my bloody bandages. She wept as she asked, "Dr. Roedde, why are you working?" An hour later, I spoke with the pathologist in Timmins, who determined that, yes, it was definitely cancer, possibly invading lymphatics (too complicated to explain, but not good). I asked my receptionist if the nurse or nurse practitioner could take my last patient. Then I went off to the local Catholic church to pray.

I declined chemo. How would I explain why I was puking and bald? I was having a hard enough time recovering from the surgery. Twice a week, a huge, blood-filled haematoma in my breast was drained by my surgeon, Dr. Rahn. I did not know him as well as I knew Jake, which made this intimate invasion easier. In late fall, I met Vicki in Sudbury, the day I had a breast surgeon assess that same large haematoma, my blood leaking into my bra. I had bought a new bra and new sweater to replace the blood-stained ones. She was wise and comforting. "You'll get through this, Gretch! We're all with you."

By Christmas I had driven three hours to Sudbury on a treacherous ice-filled highway for a diagnosis by sentinel-node biopsy of my lymph nodes, to confirm that the cancer had not spread. And after singing in the French Catholic choir for midnight Mass, I was back in Sudbury getting small pin-point tattoos on my chest to guide the radiation. I was freaking out over the permanent disfiguration by scar and tattoos. Five weeks of radiation followed, when I learned how to nap. I took up knitting again. The Sudbury Cancer Centre has baskets of knitting for patients and their friends; you knit however many rows you have time for while waiting for appointments and radiation treatments. There is a small ruler, and whoever knits to the required size casts off the piece. These squares are then knitted together to form afghans for the beds we slept in at the residence for cancer patients, Daffodil Terrace.

During my radiation treatments, Alec had another complication in his health, so I doubled up my treatments to two a day, to look after him in hospital.

When my treatments were over, I got a triumphant tattoo of a brown-eyed Susan on my left shoulder, the side of the breast cancer, to celebrate coming through. Mae and Vicki, my friends from Bear Island and godmothers to my children, kept checking in. Mae explained, "Gretchen, you have been a healer, but you need to be open to healing energy, too. You have to take time to rest. Think of the bear as an animal totem for your family. *Makwa* is Ojibwe for bear. This period of illness could be looked at as a vision quest, a time of going inward to allow the healing energy to work."

Gary Potts came over and played guitar with Alec, who was also recovering from illness. They played Alec's songs and Johnny Cash tunes. I thought of the bear that hibernates, spending time on an inward journey. I thought of Gary, who had first led us into that journey on Lake Temagami, working with his Ojibwe community, and how he had helped me understand the ending of my marriage. He had said then, "Jim and Gretchen, you were there on the threshold of our decolonization. You were inside our circle, and that is not a small thing. I am haunted by my ancestors. I am in their tents. I have to stop sometimes; the memories of all those generations are heavy. I have shared that vision with you."

These Indigenous mentors were helping my family on a journey with few signposts. I felt the way I had when I first learned to drive an open steel boat and looked around at the islands and shores full of trees, and I had asked Mae Katt, "How do you learn the way? All the islands and trees look the same. How do you find your way in the dark, in the rain?" She had shown me the patterns in trees and the land. She had shown how the shapes are different. So now our family was learning to navigate on different deep waters, in the depths of illness.

125

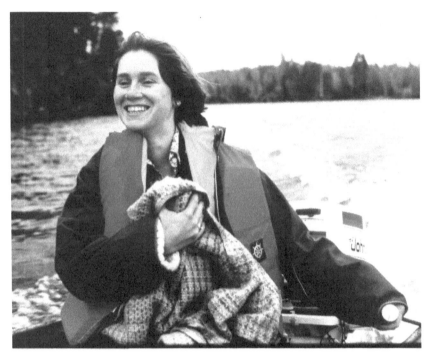

Travelling with Anna in an open steel boat, Lake Temagami, 1979.

Makwa. Bear Island. My family's life is rooted there. Years later, our strength comes from the people we are connected with. We carry that totem spirit within us. When we fall, the Bear carries us.

~ 12 ~

A GRACE-FILLED FALL

Alec recovered well from his head injury. He lived with me for many years before moving into his own home. When he had been with me for a few months, he started to plan the creation of a band. Trouble was, all his music equipment was at his dad's. Imagine my surprise when I woke at five in the morning to find a note on my kitchen table, "Gone to Winnipeg, back soon."

I went out to the garage, which was empty. At six o'clock, my hands and voice shaking, I phoned a friend who is an OPP officer. "I think my son has gone to Winnipeg. In my car. He had a recent head injury. I'm not sure how well he is to drive. What should I do?" She explained that the OPP and Manitoba police could be on the look-out for the car and stop him and ask him to phone home. At seven o'clock, I phoned Jim, who said he did know that Alec was coming to Winnipeg, though he hadn't said a word to his dad about borrowing my car.

At seven thirty that morning, I phoned his doctor, who, without violating patient confidentiality, reassured me that he thought Alec could handle this journey. The next day, Alec called to say he had arrived safely and would stop in to see Mae Katt on the way home. A few days later, he returned with a car full of amplifiers and guitars. A half hour later, his newly created band was playing in the basement.

Alec was fortunate to have many supports for his music. A short time later, Eddy and his wife, Syl, came for their first visit. In addition to being our landlord when we lived in Liverpool, Eddy was a professional composer and musician and had toured the world with his band for decades. He never travelled without a guitar.* As I drove them to our home, the blue night sky was alive with the northern lights. When we arrived at the house, Eddy stood out in the backyard to gaze wordlessly at the flashing pink and white and green flourishes of light as they cascaded across the sky. He called out, "Hey, Al, bring your guitar out here. Let's play under these northern lights." Ed pulled out his own, and the two of them stayed out playing for an hour, bouncing riffs off each other, improvising, and laughing till the transatlantic jet lag hit Ed full on and sent him to bed.

Anna came down the next morning for a grand reunion. She'd spent the summer she turned sixteen with Ed and Syl and had returned to Liverpool every year since. After kissing them both hello, she and Syl caught up on the latest Liverpool news and how the girls were doing, and Eddy and Alec headed back outside.

Eddy kept asking Alec to repeat phrases.

"Try that again, but slow it down. Sing that bit more slowly. Really emphasize the lyrics."

Ed and Syl wanted to see a First Nation community, so Alec played chauffeur when we travelled to Bear Island, down the mine road. We had borrowed an open steel boat, and Alec was now the boat expert, explaining where Gary lived as we drove by, past the band office. Alec answered Eddy's questions. "Gary used to be the Chief here, when my parents lived here with Anna. He's always been part of our family. I go to him when I'm unsure of my path."

---

*Eddy had been a long-time professional guitar player, composer, and singer. He'd started up a British-born band in Liverpool 8, a poor and largely black district. He toured internationally with his band, The Real Thing, until he died while visiting family in Australia in early 2018.

Our guests were puzzled. "So, I don't understand, mate. Where are all the teepees, wigwams, whatever you call them? Why aren't the people wearing feather headdresses?

Anna and Alec tried to explain that First Nations people live in homes like ours, some in smaller Indian Affairs regulation styles, simply and cheaply built with similar styles to each other.

"But the people don't look much different? I thought Aboriginal people here in Canada would look different, like Aboriginal people in Australia where our daughter lives."

By the end of the week, Alec was playing guitar all day, and each time we heard a new version of a song, we marvelled at how he was continually improving. (The next month, Eddy sent Alec a four-track from England, so he could record himself and listen and improve on his own.)

The following week our good friend and our son's namesake, Alex Spence, arrived from Timmins. Alex had worked with me years before on the Cree medical dictionary and was there to work at the courthouse as a justice of the peace. "How's your son doing?" he asked. He had known about Alec's times in hospital. I was excited to share the news of his progress.

Alec and Alex spent an hour talking over a supper of goose while I busied myself in the kitchen. His Cree accent was like a personal history. I remembered hearing those rich inflections from our work decades ago, in Timmins and in Fort Albany. I remembered meeting Alex in the summer of 1974, the year this professional life began. It was so rich to have a friendship with such deep roots.

My son drove our friend back to his hotel. When Alec returned, he spoke quietly. "I'm meeting Alex Spence tomorrow at sunrise. We're having a ceremony. For healing. Can I borrow the car? I'll be back before you need to leave for work."

Sure enough, he was up early and out the door. I got coffee ready for his return and made pancakes and bacon. An hour later, he came home subdued. He ate without saying much. I didn't ask him anything. I figured he'd speak to me when he was ready.

"Mom? Alex told me about the bear and helped me understand about illness. I went inside myself. Like hibernating. Now I can come back out and have the strength of that long sleep inside me. We did some smudging. I'm going to do that every day now, on my own. I burn sweetgrass, and I use this Eagle feather to waft the smoke. It purifies and heals. I'm ready now, Alex says."

CEDAR GROUNDING

I, too, was ready for healing. I was tired of patients' illnesses and of my own.

Vicki Grant called and asked if I wanted to take a sailing holiday in the Caribbean. She and Dick, and our friends David and Kathy Ramsay, who were also experienced sailors, were keen. The plan was to rent a large boat that could easily sleep the five of us. We would sail in the Grenadines for ten days.

Kathy started to look at flights while David and Dick looked into the kind of boat we might consider. I thought my ability to pack my belongings into one carry-on bag for a global health jaunt would serve me well; I'd bring a few bathing suits and T-shirts and shorts in a soft bag that could be easily stowed on a sailboat.

I remembered living with Dick and Vicki on our cedar-covered island and how, decades later, we were still so close. We'd cooked for each other and helped each other through good as well as hard times. David and Kathy had been the first friends we had made in Haileybury and New Liskeard, when the doctor who had delivered Anna invited all of us to his home. The Ramsays and the Grants had either come to my home for meals or invited me and the kids to their places in the country that was surrounded by cedars. David and Kathy had visited us at the cottage at Manitoulin Island and had taken us sailing on their boat.

I thought this trip would be a fitting way to reconnect with my own roots — my grandfather had been a sailboat designer and had spent much of his life on the water. I was recovering from breast cancer and was eager to let the sun tan the rest of my body to match my radiation burn.

I loaded up a small cloth bag with summer wear and murder mysteries. I scorn the idea of hats or sunscreen, but my daughter convinced me to bring a tube of lip gloss that had some sun protection in it — enough for my nose.

We all met at Pearson Airport, in Toronto. There were a few worried moments when Dick and Vicki were late. It was exciting to load into a plane that was not headed to a war-torn country. I could get used to this. A vacation! This was a concept I hoped to get better at, with practice.

We had a few plane changes and finally arrived in Grenada at dusk. I was charmed by the gingerbread cut-outs on the pastel-coloured buildings. We travelled by taxi to the hotel at the marina from where we would set off the next day. Outside, the crickets and frogs sang us to sleep.

In the morning we breakfasted in the open air, luxuriating in a courtyard surrounded by bougainvillea, which dropped orange, pink, and white blossoms beside our table. After breakfast we three women did a quick provisioning of the boat (Hurricane Ivan had recently passed through, and eggs were almost impossible to find, but we managed) while the men had a technical briefing of the boat's mechanical features, as well as safety precautions and the navigation systems. We loaded up the boat, making sure no cardboard boxes came aboard (they can carry eggs of pests). Then we were off!

Grenada is nestled in beautiful turquoise waters. Kathy and I went to the bow to pull up anchor. A strong current picks up shortly after you leave the harbour en route to Carriacou, several hours away. Kathy was seasick almost immediately; I had thought to take a couple of Gravol tablets. Vicki went below to organize the living quarters, and I stayed up on deck with the men, thrilled by the waves, the sun, and the huge steering wheel.

It was a long six hours on that first crossing to Carriacou. Sailing north up the Windward Islands of the Grenadines involves several passages between a chain of islands. The sea rolled the boat. I was exhilarated to sit up in the cockpit, wearing a hooded rain slicker, feeling the salt spray kiss my face. The winds were intense. Huge grey-blue breakers cascaded across the bow. Off to the starboard side, dozens of silvery fish flew across the waves pursued by an invisible predator below the surface, skimming like skipping stones flung by an unseen hand.

Fluffy pewter clouds bruised the sky above, a light rain misted over us, and above our port bow a triumphant rainbow soared across the darkening sky. I felt grateful to be alive, to feel the lightening of my own load. Sleep came quickly as we tossed gently in the bay at Carriacou, swaying on our anchor, listening to the deep sighing of the sea.

Our next crossing took us to Mayreau. We arrived at Salt Whistle Bay, a curved stretch of beach with coconut palms overhead. They provided the same sense of safety I'd had surrounded by cedars in my different Northern Ontario homes. A small dinghy came to greet us, a local man holding high a large crayfish, offering to make us a beach barbecue that evening. "Hello, my name is William. We can make you a feast! See this lobster! We have mahi-mahi, too. Freshly prepared for you this night, a picnic under the stars." We selected a mixed grill of fish, lobster, and roasted vegetables. We stayed on the boat for our sundowner, a petit punch — dark rum, demerara sugar, and limes. The sun grew heavy, slid slowly, melting along the horizon and slipping from orange to red to molten violet as it sank, the merest green flash before it left us with the darkening sky.

We clambered into our own dinghy, setting off with a small outboard to cross to the beach. We were all barefoot, nothing to hamper us as we climbed out of the boat into the salty sea. We towed the boat up onto the shore, feeling the sand between our toes, and carefully made our way over to a small picnic table. We had brought two bottles of wine, one red and one white, and five plastic glasses. Pouring out our wine, we toasted each other and our voyage.

William served us our food — steaming platters rich with the smell of land and sea. Slowly the stars came out, sparkling there above us. Small limes flavoured our fish and grilled lobster, and the vegetables had been steamed with onions and garlic. Someone mentioned Jim. I started to weep and stumbled up from my bench seat to hurry away along the beach. David caught up with me and stayed by my side as I returned to the group. It had all seemed too much. My cancer, Alec's injury, my responsibility to my patients, my sense I was doing this all alone. But I was not alone. Here with these caring friends, I was surrounded by support.

Saturday found us moored off Union Island. Vicki and I decided we would go to Mass the next day. Two young men neared our boat with a small dinghy, holding up live lobsters. "Fresh lobster? For dinner on the boat?" Once again, we arranged to savour the gifts of the sea, this time watching the sunset from our own boat as we enjoyed our evening drinks and the smell of the garlic butter and lime, while the lobster grilled on our barbecue.

In the morning, we went ashore in the dinghy. The men would explore while Vicki and I went to Mass, hiring a taxi to take us past the clapboard houses of the town to the west of the island, where a small church sat nestled in the trees. I was reminded of going to Mass with Vicki at Bear Island, in St. Ursula's church. Here, too, was a community of all ages, everyone in their Sunday best. Gradually, the congregation started to still, children no longer squirming in their seats, some, it seemed, there with their grandmothers. One of these women smiled at Vicki, her brown eyes sparkling. Though darker, she reminded me of Vicki's mother and grandmother. I thought of the webs of faith that can hold people together in difficult times. I am sure that the woman had lost loved ones, hopes, perhaps a marriage. But she was carrying on, caring for a granddaughter, I supposed, the young girl, maybe aged ten, who sat beside her. I, too, could learn to do this, to carry on.

As our voyage continued, I savoured my growing strength and healing and returned to my northern cedar-surrounded home feeling more resilient. And again I remembered my dream: the eagle flying overhead, meeting a mate, and nesting in a cold and wild grey-and-green place.

And I knew where I was on that journey after the years of slow growth and stillness, an eagle taking its own path and flying south, surrounded by warm tropical colours.

⌒

Years later, as afternoon merged with evening, I walked into another yard filled with cedars. I was visiting a new patient who I did not know well. I had met her two years earlier, when I was briefly replacing her local physician. I had learned then that she was francophone Catholic. In Northern Ontario, in Haileybury, where I live, we speak a mixture of English and French, "Franglais." About 40 percent of our community is Francophone. She told me at that appointment that when she got very sick, she wanted the support of her church. She had dressed up for that visit to see me in the clinic, with earrings and a necklace matching her brightly coloured blouse and simple tailored suit.

The doorbell did not ring, and no one answered my worried knocks on the door. I hesitated to just walk into this home I had never visited before, but Lynn, the chemo nurse, had called me to tell me the patient had not come to chemo, which was not like her. She had been valiantly struggling, requiring blood transfusions after most treatments when her counts fell too low. I opened the door, calling out, "Marie-France?" Several cats rushed to the door, hoping to sneak through. Then I heard an irritated-sounding, youthful male voice calling out to me, "Shut the door, *properly*, so the cats don't get out."

A young man rushed impatiently down the stairs, to do a better job of the door-shutting than I had managed. Marie-France was lying on the sofa bed, three Sphynx cats, hairless and narrow faced, nestled in her arms. My patient spoke feebly. "Maurice, this is Dr. Roedde."

An angry reply followed. "I don't care who she is. She should learn to shut the door."

"I didn't go to chemo today," she explained. "I'm sorry if it worried you and Lynn. I think I'm going to take a break from the chemo until I feel stronger."

That was fine with me. I had seen her in clinic a few times in the previous two months, and it was clear to me she was dying. I had already had a run-in by phone and fax with her chemo specialist at the cancer centre in Sudbury over why we were, to my mind, prolonging her suffering.

I gently nudged aside the cats intertwined on her lap, so I could listen to her chest with my stethoscope.

"We're hoarders," Maurice joked, as he stepped into the cramped living room. "I collect things and then sell them on eBay." Maurice was a single man who had decided to live at home and look after his mother, so he was able to make a little money with his collecting. Antique plates topped a sideboard and various china dolls were standing along one wall.

Every few minutes, Maurice would pop out to the back porch to have a smoke. Marie-France was wearing a simple nightdress with an open neck that allowed me to listen to her heart with my stethoscope. I noted her pulse was rapid and irregular — damage to the heart muscle from the chemo causing atrial fibrillation? Twice when I was there, Marie-France stared off vacantly into space for a few minutes and made some subtle jerking movements of her arms. Mini strokes? Or had her cancer spread to the brain?

I returned to her home that evening. Whatever was happening in her brain and the rest of her body was killing her. Maurice had been trying to get a hospital bed so she would be more comfortable, and once we got home care involved, the bed was set up in her living room. The nurse and personal support workers helped with daily visits to make sure her cancer symptoms were well managed.

Over the next four weeks, I got better at shutting the door. Marie-France had been ill for twelve years with cancer, which had started in her breast and slowly devoured her body, requiring three hospitalizations for intensive chemo and radiation treatments. She had been going weekly to the day medicine room at our local hospital, while living at home. This current cycle of palliative chemo was shrinking the tumours in her lungs, liver, bones, and adrenal glands, but she was weak and frail. She could barely stand. The skin on her arms hung loose. Her face was grey, but her smile and her brown eyes remained cheerful.

As she got too ill to walk to the washroom, and then again to get up to the commode, the family — her two sons, Maurice and Luc, and visiting sisters — used diapers to manage the incontinence as she was too restless for a catheter. Sometimes she was "there" and sometimes she wasn't. She would joke, "Dr. Roedde, now I know you are here, but in a few minutes, I will forget." The home care nurse, Dena, arrived a few minutes after me. Family and health care workers would write notes to each other on how Marie-France had been. Dena mentioned my visit after reading the notes. "Oh no," Marie-France countered, "Dr. Roedde hasn't been in." Marie-France had simply forgotten.

It had been her sixty-first birthday. She was just a few months older than me. It made me anxious to see her. Was I going to be dying at home in a few years from breast cancer, spreading and eating through my body? I, too, was being treated for breast cancer and was now taking hormonal treatments after my radiation. But Marie-France had been sick four years longer than me. I didn't want to think about that. Right now I was the doctor and she was the patient. I could not afford to identify with her. I struggled to find some way to detach myself; to not care so much about her or worry about my own health.

Sitting there in their living room, looking at Marie-France, who seemed to fade away more each day, I asked Maurice how he was doing. "This must be tough. It's hard work to watch someone as they die slowly. What can I do to help? I, too, feel powerless, as her doctor."

Maurice asked if I had a *chapelet*. "My mom is a Catholic. Maybe we can help bring her more spiritual comfort."

I brought the rosary the next day; I had bought it in Rome, at the Vatican, and it was made from wood from the Holy Land. "*C'est un cadeau pour ta fête*," I said to Marie-France, speaking in my limited French. When I had first met her two years earlier, she explained that she did not go to Mass; with her low white count from the chemo, she was worried about seeing so many people who might have coughs or colds. But she had also requested that once she got very ill, she wanted a priest to come to her home.

Dena called me at ten o'clock one night. "Dr. Roedde, she's not responsive. Maurice has just called. I told him I would meet you at the house."

I lived one town over, and twenty minutes later Dena and I, and both her weeping sons, gathered at her bed. Maurice asked, "Can you get the priest?" I phoned the nearest French Catholic church, back in Haileybury, where I sing in the choir, and the Congolese priest answered. *"Laisse-moi le temps pour ma chemise."* I picked him up twenty minutes later and drove him back to the house.

We entered, carefully shutting the door, and went through to the cluttered living room. Abbé Alexis is tall. He brings the strengths of watching life and death in an African village to his work with communities and families he ministers to in our own country. He had books of prayers, he had holy water, he had chrism, or holy oil, and he had a cross he had cherished for years, which he used to comfort the sick.

He spoke in both English and French. Marie-France had now been in a coma for two hours, and her breathing was ragged — Cheyne-Stokes, which heralds imminent death. Abbé Alexis blessed Marie-France, her sons who were caring for her, the nurse, and the doctor — *l'infirmière* and *le médecin*. His dark elongated fingers made a cross on her forehead. He led us in prayer, in French and English, "Hail Mary, full of grace." He gave me his small leather-covered book of psalms. I read Psalm 23, The Lord Is my Shepherd.

> "The Lord is my Shepherd, I shall not want.
> He makes me lie down in green pastures;
> He leads me beside still waters;
> He restores my soul. He leads me in right paths For His
> Name's sake."

I thought back to my own periods of healing, guidance, and support, sailing with friends in the Grenadines after my own time of sickness.

Maurice and his brother, Luc, each caressed their mother's hands. Their silent tears slowed. Their weeping quietened. The room became very still.

Then Marie-France opened her eyes and stared at me and then looked away, at Luc and Maurice. She gripped their hands and began speaking to them in French. It was now after midnight. I whispered to her sons that I would be back after taking the priest home. I thought she might slip away after this lucid interval, and I would need to be nearby, to pronounce her death and sign the death certificate. When I returned half an hour later, she was still talking with her sons. They knew to call me at home if she passed away in the night.

But Marie-France lived another ten days. Sisters came to see her from out west and down south. She would drift in and out of consciousness, allowing me time to call the bank to help make sure her sons would be able to keep paying the mortgage on her house from her account and giving the family a chance to get a lawyer who did a house call to arrange power of attorney and a will. Those ten days gave her time to say her goodbyes, make peace with her God, and finish the business of living. With each visit, I saw that she was slowly fading away. Frail, thin, blue-veined hands loosely clasped the rosary, holding it next to the faded quilted coverlet on the bed. The three sleek Sphynx cats were nestled in the coverlet as well, looking up at her questioningly. She lay fitfully, eyes closed, lids fluttering. She had been a thin, proud woman, neatly dressed for chemo treatments, but her skin now stretched over bone. The mottling began; the ragged breathing continued. Sometimes she would speak and look far beyond us; words that could not be understood, not in French or English, a worried murmuring. Her mouth was dry. The glycerin swabs did not help, nor did the sips of water. The lips were cracking. A bed sore had just started.

Maurice called me after midnight, one month from that first house call. "Dr. Roedde? It's Maurice. My mom has passed. It was peaceful. She just slipped away."

My final house call was calm. Marie-France was at rest, her *chapelet* gathered into her left hand. Her cheeks were cooling. Her sons and I touched her lined face. I stayed with the family till two in the morning, completing the death certificate and making sure the sons were all right. I called the funeral home, who would not be able to come to collect the body until two thirty.

Maurice smiled sadly. "It's okay, Dr. Roedde. We're okay. You don't have to wait."

I left and went home to sleep; clinic would be starting soon.

Two days later, a huge arrangement of spring flowers arrived from Maurice and Luc: pussy willows, pale purple and blue irises, pink tulips, green leaves — hopeful blossoms. When I read the card thanking me, I wept. How could they thank me? What had I given them? Had I been so moved by this family because I had this same illness? Was it my own fear of death, my own hope that there is a deeper meaning to life and to illness? I wept and I thanked them. And I thanked Marie-France.

⌒ 14 ⌒

A JUBILANT BIRTH

It was hard to spend so much time with the dying. But I liked providing care in people's homes. Years after my own early training with the midwives in the U.K., I was able to renew that great first love and celebrate a jubilant birth in my home.

Now past sixty years of age, I was working full-time in a clinic in Latchford, a town twenty minutes south of my home. Alec was living around the corner with his girlfriend, Hayley, in his sister's former house. I had last delivered a baby in a pickup truck in Tanzania, when our health team had given a lift to a man who was carrying his labouring wife in a basket on his bike. The week before I left for that assignment, I had done a few deliveries with one of our local GPs who did a lot of obstetrics —"Just in case I end up doing a delivery when I'm in Africa."

Since starting in Latchford, I was much more involved with our local hospital staff and had met the two midwives, Kim and Paule — lively young women with small children — one day after Grand Rounds. This is a happy gathering of staff who always greet each other with warm grins or a hug in the boardroom once a month. "Come to our open house next week!" the midwives said, with huge smiles. Paule and Kim spoke English to me but French with each other.

I thought this would be a great idea. I had things I could share: flashcards on warning signs in labour and delivery for less literate health workers from my work travels abroad; training manuals for traditional birth attendants in countries where doctors are seldom available. We talked about my work in various countries with maternity waiting homes where rural women can come before delivery, and about the problems of health financing to overcome the barriers of user pay health systems, which penalize poor women. Except for those local deliveries, all the births I had been involved with since med school had taken place in barns with the water buffalo in Nepal, in small rooms with roosters in Bangladesh, and in mud huts in various African countries.

At the open house, Kim and Paule shared their concerns about the Amish and Mennonite women who lived a couple of hours away from our hospital. Kim explained that typically these communities do not participate in our national funded health system but pay cash for services such as blood work, ultrasounds, or hospital birthing. "We're salaried, so our services are available to them. The Amish are very family-centred, and most women have six or more children. They're such gentle women and prefer to deliver at home. They wear their grey handmade clothes and bonnet even when they give birth. But we're worried about doing home deliveries that far from hospital. You know how often the highway is closed in the winter."

Paule agreed. "We have delivered in very simple rooms with no windows or lights. We don't know if there is placenta previa.* An ultrasound to detect this is not often done because it costs a few hundred dollars. We don't know if the woman might start to bleed. We bring IVs and medicines for hemorrhage, but if there is a placenta previa those are not enough to keep the woman from bleeding to death. It would be over an hour to get to the hospital where we can get a Caesarean section. We let the paramedics know when we are doing a home birth and give them our location, but our cellphones don't always work. There is rarely good

---

*This is where the placenta is positioned before the baby and is attached to the lower part of the uterus so there is hemorrhage during the delivery, and a Caesarean section is needed to save both mother and baby.

lighting, even though we bring battery-operated suction and resuscitation equipment for the newborn."

Kim nodded. "We rent space in a local health facility for pre-natals but aren't allowed to do deliveries there. If we can't do a home birth at a woman's own residence, we have to take her to hospital, at her expense if she is not covered by OHIP (Ontario Health Insurance Plan, or Medicare) because of the community's religious beliefs opposing social insurance. We have two women who are due in February."

I was excited to have a local bridge to my global health work. "Your stories remind me so much of my overseas work where the midwives deliver women with candles in their teeth so they can see and keep their hands free. Why had the health system not made battery-operated headlamps available to midwives for deliveries in poor countries that usually had no electricity and few drugs? I would love to talk about all this again. Come to my house next," I invited them. "Let's have lunch and see where it leads us."

I live in a large prairie-yellow house, fronted by a wide, winterized porch full of windows. It has five bedrooms. I live there with two ginger cats.

Paule came with French onion soup, Kim brought a huge salad, and I provided juice and white wine for our lunch. We toured my house, full of light and stained glass windows I have made. When we reached my sewing room upstairs, Paule took one look at the long built-in desk and cupboards on one side and exclaimed, "This would be perfect for a birthing room! See, here we can resuscitate the baby, the woman can labour and deliver on this futon, and we can keep our supplies in the cupboards!"

I must admit, this thought had never occurred to me. I have a lot of hobbies, and as my children were grown up, the bedrooms had been converted into studios — a weaving studio, stained glass/mosaic tile studio, the sewing room, a study for writing. Bright sunlight streamed in through the windows and filtered warmly against the peach-coloured walls. I decided to wait a bit before discussing the home insurance implications of such a venture with my agent. He was also unaware of my habit of driving on closed highways in the winter to get to work.

But it wouldn't be a business anyway, would it? The midwives could use my home as a birthing centre near the hospital if things went wrong for their Amish and Mennonite patients. I looked at it as an extension of hospitality, not as work. People often stay at my home when bad weather closes the roads. The midwives knew how to get in if I was away. "Just phone and let me know you're on your way; leave a message, but I could be anywhere." I was going out of town that weekend, so I did a rushed tidy-up of the sewing room, removing clothes from the drawers and material from the cupboards. I moved the sewing machine off the desk and shoved it into a closet in another room. A standing lamp from the porch worked well near the bed, to provide the midwives with adequate bright light. We now had the Amish birthing room.

———

One Monday in February, I returned home from a writing weekend away, driving directly from my cottage to work. My secretary called out to me as I came into the office and kicked off my boots, "Kim is on the phone for you!"

"Gretchen, we're at your place. Our patient is just four centimetres. It'll be a while yet. She did get an ultrasound a few weeks ago, and she's overdue, forty-one weeks, but her contractions are still irregular."

I had patients in clinic that morning and medical students at the hospital in the afternoon. "I'll swing by at noon and see how everyone is getting on."

At lunch, I drove to my home, the new birthing centre. It seemed strange to walk into my house as a somewhat respectful outsider. Two pairs of black boots, one larger for a man and one smaller for his wife, stood at my entryway. Two dark hats, the taller for the husband and a smaller outer bonnet for his wife, were laid carefully on the shelf over the radiator by the door. I threw my coat over the bannister and tentatively went up the stairs. I tiptoed into the stained-glass studio, where

144

Paule was stretched out on a white wicker chair; Ginger, the cat with the marmalade fur, was curled up in her lap. Paule was reading the discharge summary from her patient's previous delivery.

"Gretchen, hello! I'm just going to check on Hannah. Come and meet her husband, Christian. Hannah is resting. Labour hasn't progressed much. The baby's heart rate has been good, though. I was thinking I might break her waters."

Paule got up and opened the glass French doors separating the stained-glass studio from the weaving studio. Two brightly painted tapestries cover the doors for privacy. Christian, with a long beard and mutton chops, and wearing blue trousers with suspenders and a lighter blue long-sleeved shirt, was seated on a white wicker chair. Paule introduced us. Christian stood and nodded, putting his newspaper and bag of potato chips to the side. As he was reading, automatically I went to turn on the overhead light, but he gestured there was no need; he had opened the blinds so the room was filled with natural light. I remembered that the Amish seldom use electricity. I wasn't sure of the proper etiquette. Many traditional cultures limit physical contact between men and women who do not know each other. Does one shake hands? Nod and smile? I opted for the latter.

"Christian," continued Paule, "we're just going to check on Hannah. Is that okay?"

"Yes, yes, fine," he murmured.

The Amish don't own cars and share a communal phone, which is housed in an outbuilding. They have non-Amish friends they can get lifts from and whose phones they can use. Christian had called Paule early in the morning; she had met them in the centre of town and driven with them to my home.

Paule and I entered my sewing room, the birthing centre. Hannah was standing in her white bonnet and long grey dress. "I'm just going to check you. Is it okay if Dr. Roedde is here?"

"Yes, sure," said Hannah in a slight German accent, smiling sweetly.

Hannah lay down on the bed. Paule gloved up and checked her. "Still just four centimetres. Let me see if I can break your waters and move things along." Paule had what looked like a hanging garment bag full of pockets: hooks to break the waters, suturing materials, gloves, medications for bleeding and infection, and clamps for the cord, all neatly labelled. She spoke in a calm voice, reassuring Hannah by explaining everything she was doing. She tried three times to break the waters, but to no avail. Later, after Hannah delivered, the midwives discovered that the placenta was almost calcified because the birth was overdue; when the membranes finally ruptured, there was no amniotic fluid, but the placenta was still soft enough to deliver easily. "I'm just going to check the baby. Are you having a contraction?"

Paule put her hand on Hannah's belly, feeling the strength of the contraction. When the tightening eased off, Paule checked the fetal heart with her Doppler, a small hand-held instrument that amplifies the sound of the baby's heartbeat. The heart rate had dropped to 80 per minute. After a minute, it came back up to 120. "Let's try to change your position. Maybe the baby isn't getting enough blood flow because you're lying on your back, and there is too much pressure on a large blood vessel there. Let's try you standing up." Again, Paule checked Hannah when she was standing, just after the contraction and then a few minutes later. Each time the heart rate dropped to 80, then came back up to 120. "I'm going to send a message to my colleague, Kim," Paule explained to Hannah. "She's on her way."

A few minutes later, Kim came up the stairs and they discussed the situation. Paule rechecked the fetal heartbeat so Kim could also hear. "Yes, the heart rate keeps dropping, even with a change of position. And she's still only four centimetres dilated. I don't like that, so early in the labour. Hannah, you know what we had discussed? If we think you would be safer in the hospital? Let's talk to Christian." The midwives explained that they thought Hannah needed to be in hospital. "We know this is costly for you. But it's safer for Hannah and the baby. That is why we're in Dr. Roedde's house, as it's only a short drive away."

Christian turned to his wife. "What do you want? Whatever you want."

Hannah wanted the safety of the hospital, and I continued to be moved by how attentive Christian was to her wishes.

I knew Kim and Paule were fine. One would drive and one would attend Hannah on the way. I left to teach my students, also up at the hospital. I could check in after my class finished at four thirty.

I had exciting news for my five students, that my first visitors to the Amish birthing centre were en route. Another three students joined us by video conference hookup; our class flew by. We had been discussing labour and delivery and resuscitation of the newborn, so this was very complementary. At the end of the session, I rushed over to the OB ward, where Paule met me, wearing her greens.

"The O.R. docs were all prepped for a Caesarean section. She was still only four centimetres and kept having the decelerations. We had two GP-OB docs, including Dr. Desilets, and a GP anaesthetist check as well. Dr. Percy was here to do an IV, and Dr. Currie was ready to do the C-section. We were just transferring her to the stretcher to take her into the O.R. when she started really strong contractions and dilated quickly. She delivered vaginally! At two twenty-five p.m., less than an hour after leaving your place! The cord was wrapped around the neck, which is probably why the heart rate kept dropping."

A smiling Paule led me to the labour room, where Hannah was resting comfortably with her new baby girl in her arms. "It was good we had come to your home. Thank you so much. We really appreciate what you've done. I'll tell my sister Clara. She's due this week!"

I failed to keep the tears from welling up in my eyes. Why did I try to hide them? I used to cry after every delivery I did during my internship.

I spent a few minutes talking with Christian and explained that I would like to meet with the Elders of the community, to better understand why they did not participate in Medicare. I was concerned about these costs they had to pay — for the ultrasound, the hospital care. The next morning, I met with the hospital accountants to see what the family might expect to pay for the hospital birth. I agreed to follow up with our hospital and other local hospitals that have Amish and Mennonite patients who "pay direct." There had to be a way to offer reduced fees. As in my work overseas, ethnic minority people have more trouble accessing medical services and have lower rates of skilled attendance at delivery, so it felt right to be doing the same kind of work here.

On Wednesday night my son Alec and his partner, Hayley, came for supper. As we were chatting and preparing dinner, the phone rang. Alec picked it up after a nod and a questioning raised eyebrow to me. I was turning steaks in the pan. "Mom, it's Kim, the midwife." I quickly turned off the pan and took the phone from his hand.

"Gretchen? We have another Amish woman who is close to giving birth. Maybe tomorrow?"

"Same drill," I answered. "Just leave a message and make yourselves at home."

We settled in to our supper. Hayley, in particular, was pretty excited. "I think this is very cool what you're doing."

"Are you sure I haven't lost my mind?"

"Well," she said, chuckling.

After Alec and Hayley left, I prepared the meal for the next night. At the end of a four-week module with my students, I cook them a meal. The next day I was going to facilitate our final session, give my feedback for the teleconference students, then come home to the five local students and give them each their personalized evaluation, using forms from the Northern Ontario School of Medicine, while we all had our meal and dessert. My students had different food preferences, so the menu included five split-roasted Rock Cornish game hens, a beef bourguignon, and asparagus, all prepped and placed in the breezeway to keep cool overnight.

The next day I rushed home between clinic and class after an update call from Kim. I scooted into the kitchen through the back door, noting two new pairs of dark shoes and dark hats, as well as the midwife's coat and boots. I popped my head upstairs to find Kim in the hall.

"This is Clara. She has been labouring for a few hours but is not having very regular contractions. I just broke her waters; there was lots of fluid, and she's about five centimetres. Here is her husband, Noah."

I turned and greeted him. Like Christian, he wore a light blue shirt, with darker blue suspenders, over a denim blue-coloured pair of trousers. He, too, had a beard and was gently attentive to his wife, rubbing her back whenever she had contractions.

Kim took me aside. "Looks like you're having people for dinner?"

I explained it would be the medical students, and we would remain downstairs so as not to interrupt the labouring Amish family. Kim could come and go. Again, the afternoon class passed in a whir as I wondered how Clara and Noah were getting on. I returned at four thirty and popped in my head as Kim was checking her patient. "Clara, you're still not having regular contractions, and you're only about five centimetres." I was curious; this seemed a slow progression of labour for someone who had other kids, so I asked Clara, "How many children have you had?" She smiled dreamily and told me, "I have four. The oldest is four. She is such a great help!" I thought to myself, there aren't many families I know who would consider four-year-olds as a great help.

The students arrived an hour later. We had our meal, the meats accompanied by salads, bottles of soft drinks, wine, and beer. I did the evaluations while Kim came down and chatted with the students. She told me that should Clara deliver while they were there, the three female students could observe the birth. By nine thirty that evening, the students were gone. Kim and I went up to check on Clara, whose contractions were getting stronger but were still not regular. The baby's heart rate was strong at 140 per minute and not slowing after a contraction. Kim decided not to check the cervix again for four hours. "I already know she's not having strong contractions," she explained. "As long as the heart rate is good, we're fine. No point in introducing the risk of infection."

By ten thirty, the situation was unchanged. Kim told me, "I'm just going to text the OB nurse, Becca, who was here earlier today to meet Noah and Clara, that we're going to rest, and we'll call her when things start to happen."

We spoke with the family about the plans. Kim was going to sleep in another bedroom upstairs. "Just knock on the door when the contractions get more intense," she told Clara.

I retreated to my own room downstairs, changed into leggings and a short-sleeved T-shirt, an outfit as suitable for sleep as it was to assist a delivery. At one thirty in the morning, I woke to the sound of rapid pacing upstairs along with strong, shuddering breaths. I got up, splashed some water on my face, and tiptoed upstairs just as Clara was knocking on Kim's bedroom door. Noah was rubbing Clara's back as she took deep breaths to manage the intensity of the contractions. Kim got the Doppler and declared, "We have a happy baby in there! Still 140 beats a minute."

Kim and I went into the birthing room to review the neonatal resuscitation equipment and oxygen. She sent a text message to update Becca that things were moving quickly. As Kim went to wash her hands, the light burned out overhead. I did a quick run around the house for a replacement bulb, found it, and then looked up at the bathroom ceiling, well beyond my reach. Noah came over and stood quietly beside me. "Let me help." He reached up to replace the bulb. I marvelled at the fact that this gentle Amish man, with no electricity, was calmly adapting to the situation and was willing to help me with my own electrified home.

Kim asked, "Do you want to deliver this baby standing? Like your last baby?" Clara smiled softly, her hands clasped over her rounded blue frock. "I think so. It's better for me." Many women in villages around the world know that this can make for an easier birth. Kim asked her, "Is it okay if we let Dr. Roedde do the delivery? You're my patient, and she will be working under my supervision." Clara, still holding her unborn baby, murmured, "We would be happy if she did this. We are enjoying being in her home."

Kim lay plastic sheeting and absorbent pads on the floor to catch the amniotic fluid and told me what to expect.

"Clara will be positioned like this," she said, leaning over the desk where we had the resuscitation equipment. "You sit on the futon behind her. The baby will be face-first in this position. You'll hand the baby through her legs to Becca, who will be waiting." Just then Becca arrived in the room. As she passed me, I read LIFEGUARD on the back of her red T-shirt as she took her place.

The contractions were getting stronger now, and Noah was rubbing his wife's back. Clara still wore her white bonnet and grey dress. Kim did a quick check, and the baby's head was just there but would recede between contractions. Clear fluid was still being expressed with no sign of meconium, the dark green-to-black fecal matter that is sometimes visible in the amniotic fluid, a sign of trouble to birth attendants. Becca now did a check for the baby's heart rate: 140, a regular, healthy rate. "Still a happy baby!" exclaimed Kim with a smile.

I slipped gloves on and positioned my hands over the baby's head so I could feel how much the baby was descending with each contraction and to have gentle pressure there to prevent the baby coming out too quickly, in case the cord was around the neck.

"Can I push now?" asked Clara. She hardly showed that she was in pain, even though she was in the most intense stage of labouring. She leaned over the long desk for support. "Yes, go ahead," replied Kim.

Clara pushed now with each contraction. The baby's head became more exposed. I placed my gloved hands, one below the other, over the glistening dark hair. One strong contraction came and out came the baby's face. I quickly slipped my fingers inside the cervix and around the neck to feel for the cord. Kim quickly checked as well — no cord. With the next contraction, the wet, slippery baby was in my waiting blue-gloved hands, crying with a bit of a gurgling sound.

Noah rubbed Clara's back. She was still clothed in her simple frock and sighed happily in her German-accented English, "The baby is fine?" She turned to her husband and smiled. Clara looked joyous and serene. I had never seen such a peaceful birth nor witnessed such presence and dignity in a woman delivering.

"It's a boy!" exclaimed Kim. I passed the baby through Clara's legs to Becca like some kind of football manoeuvre. She lifted him and bundled him in warm blankets. Kim and I eased Clara back onto the bed and positioned her sidesaddle, with her legs toward me. Kim handed me the cord clamps, which I first clamped on the cord close to the baby's umbilicus, then a couple of centimetres toward the placenta. "Now it's your job!" Kim said to Noah, handing him the scissors to cut the cord between the two clamps. The baby was still crying well and was warmly wrapped. We could see nice pink skin even at the feet. Clara put him on the breast; this releases the hormone oxytocin, which would help reduce her own bleeding. To add to nature's design, Becca reached over and gave Clara an injection of oxytocin in her anterior thigh, to control bleeding and help expel the afterbirth.

Becca also drew up vitamin K for the baby. Newborns are deficient in this vitamin, which protects against bleeding by helping blood to clot. Because breast milk has very little vitamin K, a shot of it protects the baby for several months against different bleeding problems. Becca injected the baby's thigh. He was nuzzling at his mother's discreetly covered breast and starting to suckle as Clara caressed his still-wet head.

"This is a big baby! Any guesses as to the weight?" Kim smiled over to Clara, who was propped up on the pillows on the bed. Noah stood beside her. Our choices were in the eight- to nine-pound range. Kim and I watched for the lengthening of the cord, the sign that the placenta was separating from the womb. I pulled slowly but firmly with a downward motion. Becca handed over the stainless steel basin (in its previous life, a large mixing bowl from my kitchen) to receive the placenta, like a large slab of liver, with the cord attached. This had nourished the baby through its development. Kim checked it over, pointing out the insertion of the cord on the side and the fact that all the membranes were intact, which meant none had been left inside Clara to cause continued bleeding.

"Let's weigh the baby," said Kim. She brought out a hanging scale and lay the baby in its pouch. "Nine pounds, twelve ounces!" Clara and Noah smiled at each other, as did Becca, Kim, and I. Becca looked at her watch. "Baby was born at three thirty a.m. I've written it down in the notes, as well as the time the placenta was delivered, and the APGARS [a numeric scale for how healthy a baby is at birth in terms of colour, muscle tone, cry, etc.]. Now I'm off because I have to be at work for seven a.m." She headed out with a cheery wave and down the stairs as we watched the red LIFEGUARD recede.

Kim checked for bleeding, which was minimal and controlled. She looked at me with a jubilant smile. "There is nothing else like it.

Nothing like bringing a new life into the world. Isn't birth a miracle? I'm going to go home to sleep for a while. I have to be up with my kids in the morning and get them fed and ready for school." She turned to Clara. "I'll be back to check on you around ten a.m."

I invited Clara and Noah to keep resting and told them I'd see them in the morning before I went to work. I walked back downstairs and then lay in my own bed, celebrating the birth.

At six thirty that morning, I got up and greeted Noah, who was on the phone arranging a ride home to do chores. I showed him how to make toast in the toaster oven and explained that there was fruit salad and juice for Clara. We both went upstairs, where Clara lay sleepily on the futon in the room where she had given birth. "I have had a rest. I am tired, but I'm okay."

Noah brought in the phone, and we both showed her how to use it in case she had heavy bleeding and needed to call Kim. I was thrilled. Cellphone averse as I am, much to the chagrin of my children, I could actually teach an Amish woman to use my portable phone in case of emergency to call the midwife. I left, exhilarated and exhausted, and went for my usual morning swim.

On my way to work, I stopped back in to check on Clara, to make sure there was no heavy bleeding and to see that she had eaten something to keep up her strength. I remembered the births of my own children, how exhausted I had been. I was all too aware of how fragile new life is and was still amazed to have played a role in delivering her baby. Clara's colour was better now, and the remains of her toast, fruit, and juice were in empty dishes on the floor beside her bed.

"I am so lucky! I don't usually get breakfast in bed!" she said. I went back downstairs to make her more. Brigid, the Scottish midwife, had taught me well.

SECTION FOUR

KEEWATINONG / key-weh-di-noong /
Spirit Keeper of the North

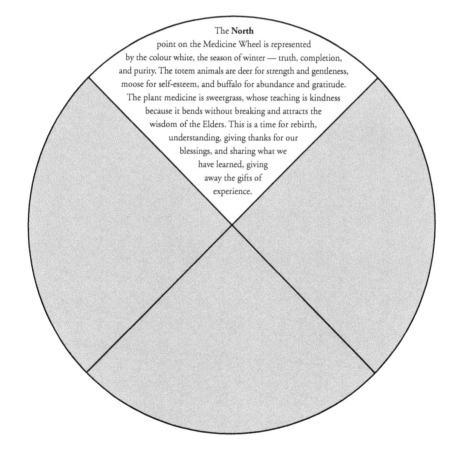

The **North**
point on the Medicine Wheel is represented
by the colour white, the season of winter — truth, completion,
and purity. The totem animals are deer for strength and gentleness,
moose for self-esteem, and buffalo for abundance and gratitude.
The plant medicine is sweetgrass, whose teaching is kindness
because it bends without breaking and attracts the
wisdom of the Elders. This is a time for rebirth,
understanding, giving thanks for our
blessings, and sharing what we
have learned, giving
away the gifts of
experience.

~ 15 ~

MOOSE ON THE
RED SQUIRREL ROAD

The leaves were all starting to turn dark rusty reds and oranges, shimmering with green. We are the northernmost limit of the maples, and we have lots of conifers. It was fall of 2012 when I got a call that a man named Ronnie Paige was coming in to talk about his most recent appointment in Sudbury. He'd had several rounds of chemo and surgery at the regional cancer centre for more than a decade. His bowel cancer had now spread to lung, liver, and bone. "They have decided there is nothing more to be done," he explained. "But I can try to see if I can get into a trial somewhere."

Ronnie was still a big guy, barrel-chested, and clean-shaven. A couple of his teeth were broken from the chemo, but he always seemed to be smiling or laughing.

We sent him to two major cancer centres in Toronto and London, Ontario, to look at drug trials, but they were too expensive and too experimental, so Ronnie decided to forego them. "Just keep me hunting and fishing for as long as possible, and let me have time with my family."

Ronnie was like a godfather to Alec's fiancée, Hayley, and I'd learned about Ronnie's love of the outdoors from her. "See, here's a picture of me when I was about six, at the hunt camp," she told me. "And here I'm a teenager, aiming a shotgun when we were hunting moose. Ronnie was one of the people who taught me to shoot. Nicky and Ronnie are like another set of parents to me."

Ronnie and his French-Canadian wife, Nicky, had raised lots of kids — two of their own, and a slew of grandkids, nieces, and nephews, as well as a few neighbourhood kids who needed some extra parenting. Hayley's own parents were best friends with Nicky and Ronnie, so Hayley was already family.

I was still working full-time in Latchford, where Hayley and her mom had both grown up. Hayley's sister-in-law was the town financial officer. Many of my patients I saw were their family and friends, making it tricky to keep boundaries professional. What's more, Ronnie's illness was not secret or private, and when I made house calls, family and friends were usually there.

Nicky was keeping his meds organized. He was okay for pain on just Percocet for hunting season, and with only a handful of pills could get out to the bush. Sometimes he would sneak various grandkids out to camp and "help" them skip school, covering for them with their parents.

That winter, Ronnie took a turn for the worse. His cancer had returned with a vengeance, and he started to have pain in his belly. A surgeon agreed he might have a bowel obstruction, but he also believed that the risks of surgery outweighed any benefits in a man with an incurable cancer.

Two days later the weather turned blizzardy, with wild drifting snow and zero visibility. As I drove carefully through the town of Cobalt, appreciating the heated seats in my all-wheel-drive Subaru Outback, I came to a sign above the road at the junction of Highway 11 and 11B that read "Highway closed at Temagami." There had been yet another accident south of Temagami at Sand Dam Road, site of so many accidents every year. Highway 11 was closed in both directions. I knew I had patients booked at the clinic in Latchford, and I had to check on Ronnie and visit other sick people at home, many of whom had no cars to get north to the emerg at the hospital in New Liskeard. In any case, if the roads were closed, I'd best go down and see how the community was faring. I needed to get to the clinic. I also needed to check on lab results of patients I had seen the previous week.

When the highways are closed, and one still goes ahead and drives on them, it's best to have a good relationship with the insurance agent and confess to bad behaviour, but for good reasons, to make sure of coverage in the case of an accident. My agent thinks I'm okay if I drive slowly and carefully. Ambulances have had to drive my patients on a closed highway to get to treatment in Timmins or Sudbury.

So I took a long, slow route, driving mindfully. Through the towns is easier, as the roads are plowed and sanded better and there aren't any police cars, because they are all busy stopping cars on Highway 11, the main road.

Highway 11 was crazy with blowing snow; I pretended to not see the barriers preventing me from driving north or south and drove around them. The roads were desolate. I felt like I was on the moon. Nothing moved in either direction. There is one advantage of driving on a closed highway. No one else was crazy enough to be on it. I inched my way forward, as I could see so little. I felt as if I were driving in a swirling talcum powder storm. My tires crunched on the frozen snow beneath me. I was grateful for my heated car — the thermostat on the dash read thirty degrees below zero as the outside temperature. What usually took ten minutes from the 11/11B cut-off took me twenty-five minutes driving blind.

I turned onto the clinic's street and popped my head into the staff entryway. "Sorry I'm late!" I shook the snow off my boots as I came in the back door to the clinic.

"Don't take off your boots!" my secretary called out, coming into the staff kitchen. "Nicky called. Ronnie is sick and you need to go see him. The first patient cancelled because she couldn't get here from New Liskeard with the closed roads, so you have time to do a house call."

Ronnie's house was nearby. As always, I parked my car in the driveway, walked past the mailbox shaped like a fish, and let myself in the front door. I took off my boots in the mudroom and walked through the kitchen in my stocking feet. Ronnie was lying in his hospital bed in the adjoining living room, and Nicky was standing in the kitchen with her sister-in-law Georgia beside her. I called, "Hello!"

"You should have just left your boots on!" chided Nicky. "Hey, have you had breakfast? Ronnie isn't eating, but we have bacon and eggs if you want."

"Let me sort out Ronnie, Nick. I'll just be a few minutes." I turned over to Ronnie, keeping my voice low so he could reply in kind and we could have a little privacy. "So, big guy, what's up?" He once had been a big guy, but now he was losing weight quickly. His face was losing its cheeky roundness. But the merry smile never changed.

Ronnie hated to complain. No matter how bad it was, you would never hear it from Ronnie. In fact, he didn't talk much but always greeted the world with a teasing smile and a quip. He had given nicknames to most of his family friends. The kids who used to go to his hunt camp always considered it an honour to get renamed by him.

"Oh, it's nothing much." His hands hung loosely at his sides as I came over to his bed to examine him. According to Nicky he was having pain, though he was not holding his abdomen.

"Come on, Ronnie, tell her!" exclaimed Nicky.

He turned away, embarrassed. "Nick, it's nothing!'

"Dr. Roedde, he hasn't passed his bowels for five days, and his belly is hurting him real bad. He feels sick to his stomach, and he vomited this morning."

His stomach was distended and tense. As I examined him gently, I saw from the grimaces that he was trying to hide his pain. His breath smelled bad, like a fart. I thought he had a bowel obstruction, and he needed to get back to our hospital to the same surgeon he had seen a couple of days earlier. I phoned up to the hospital and got Dr. Jamal Alsharif. "I think he has a bowel obstruction. Can I send him up?"

Jamal agreed. "Don't let him eat or drink, and get him up here."

There was lots of help at the house, and Ronnie's son, Chris, seemed to be always there. Chris was like an uncle to Hayley's son, Regan, always taking him hunting and fishing. It was no problem to get the truck running, warm it up, help the patient in, and assemble a couple of people to help out — someone to look after him and some-one to drive expertly on the closed highway. By that evening, Ronnie had been operated on and was resting comfortably. Two days later he was home.

———

Soon the snow was melting on the cedars and pines, and a few green shoots were coming through the previous year's brown grass. Chickadees whirled wildly in the trees, seeking out bright red mountain ash berries to eat. As spring began, Ronnie started to fail, and he was still losing weight. On many of the house calls I made, I would meet Hayley or her parents or her sister. Everyone was drawing closer in support.

One Saturday in May, I was on my way to another house call at Ronnie's, the second that day. His pain had worsened. I slowed my car right down to a stop at a stretch of Highway 11B after Mud Lake Road and before Portage Bay Road. Early green leaves were just starting to bud on the birches and poplars, appearing soft against the white and grey bark. The water was open — a recent and welcome change — and the shifting of those white ice floes to green and brown waters moved the spirit. A mother lynx and three cubs wandered sleepily across the road, oblivious to me as I slowed to a stop. She was bigger than a fox but not as tall as a wolf. The mother in the lead and the first cub had just gotten to the right side of the road; the other two cubs were waiting tentatively in the middle, looking at their mom. She looked back at them, her peaked ears alert, her grey-blue dappled coat shining in the cool spring sun. She was about twice the size of her cubs. I sat in my car for five minutes, slowing my breathing from the adrenaline of yet another distress call. I turned the motor off. Slowly the last two cubs sprinted across, and the family disappeared into the bush. I restarted the car and thoughtfully made my way over to the Paige house, which was nestled in the woods.

Cars and trucks and a motorhome of visiting family members crowded the driveway. Nicky greeted me, as always, with kind offers. "Dr. Roedde, do you want a Fudgsicle? Chips? Juice?" I declined and then snacked on one potato chip when I figured she wasn't looking.

161

Ronnie was having more pain in his abdomen. I sent him up to the hospital for a palliative care consult.

A few days later, he came home with a fentanyl narcotic patch, because he wanted to go fishing. It would serve him better than a pump, though Nicky was a bit worried. She was a trooper, ready to do whatever needed to be done for her man, the love of her life. But she wanted re-assurance. "Is he going to be okay on fentanyl patches while we take him fishing down at the camp, miles into the bush?"

The family was ready to take the risk of taking him down thirty kilometres of bad road to a place with no cellphone coverage. I gave Nicky instructions about how much extra she might need to add to the patches he was already using. It was a major family outing. Chris's wife, Angela, had just given birth to baby Ronnie and was still new to breastfeeding. I suggested that with the chaos of it all, she should bring backup formula. The truck roared down the road past the clinic with waving hands and laughing faces in the windows.

One night in August, Nicky called. Ronnie hadn't been able to pee for a day, and with his belly swollen, he was very uncomfortable. I called Kathy, the home care nurse. It was close to midnight. "I think he needs to be catheterized," I told her. "Can you go down to see him?"

Our home care nurses are outstanding. Kathy lives a half-hour north, but down she drove to Latchford late that night and got him catheterized. His pain stopped.

The trouble with catheters, though, is the risk of infection. Bladder infections can get pretty serious with sick patients. Nicky would call when the urine got red or cloudy. At the time, I had a medical student working with me. Jen was tall, with swinging shoulder-length hair, a steady smile, and quick answers to any medical question.

I asked her, "What does it mean when the urine is cloudy? What is the risk here?"

"He needs antibiotics. He could develop delirium," replied Jen.

Then I added, "Right, we'll call Findlay's pharmacy and have them delivered today. He can get septic quickly."

Ronnie would improve for a few days, then get confused and go downhill. Back I would go with Jen, who worked with me for several weeks. Gesturing to Ronnie, I explained, "See, he is confused; he's not responding. This is a delirium. We'll change the antibiotic and hope for the best."

On a day when the urine was clear, he was still having severe abdominal pain, so it seemed it wasn't an infection. The stretching of the liver kept getting worse. He was now getting pretty yellow — jaundice from the cancer spread to the liver.

Ronnie was having trouble sleeping, and he took a variety of medicines for that — oxazepam, lorazepam, and such. Nicky was also finding it hard to cope, and she required sleeping meds, too. Some days were stressful for everyone, watching a strong man struggle with such severe illness and pain. Nicky would joke, "What would be the dose of lorazepam for my nephew? My grandson? The dog? We're all going to need them."

It reached the point when it was time to switch Ronnie to a pain pump, which would allow the narcotic (in this case, hydromorphone) to be infused into Ronnie's body via a "subcu line." *Subcutaneous* means under the skin. With this method of administration, the medication doesn't go into a vein but, rather, is injected into the tissue layer between the skin and the muscle. Once the line is installed, the patient can just push a button when they need a top-up of pain medication. The preset limit can be increased as the pain progresses.

Ronnie was thrilled. "Hey, why didn't we think of this before?"

"Remember? You thought the patch would be easier for fishing!"

Two weeks later, on a Sunday, Nicky called again. "Ronnie can't move his legs. Can you come down?" By this point, we were expecting him to live just a few weeks if we were lucky. I was pretty worried. I drove down to Latchford, feeling sad. Sure enough, Ronnie could not move his legs, and the pain in his back was intense. We increased the setting on his pain pump. I knew the cancer had spread into his spine and was affecting the spinal cord. He was already unable to move his bowels or pass urine on his own. Now he was paralyzed below the waist. He would have to go to Sudbury for radiation to try to shrink the tumour and help reduce the bone pain. "Will I be able to walk again after the radiation?"

"Ronnie, let's just take this day by day. First we have to get you more pain relief."

I left the family, with Nicky waving cheerily to me. "Dr. Roedde, you know where we keep the key to the house. Any time you need a place to stay!"

I drove over to the clinic and wrote up a referral for palliative radiation in Sudbury to shrink the tumour and faxed it off. The next morning, the Sudbury hospital replied that they could take him as soon as he could get there. A one-day response time in Northern Ontario for palliative radiation!

When you have a Home Care pain pump, ambulances are not allowed to transport you to hospital. Sudbury is about two and a half hours by road, if you're driving quickly. It's longer going the speed limit with a patient aboard.

On Monday morning, Ronnie's wife, son, and nephew Randy helped load him into the truck. There was always an RV in the driveway or yard. Nicky's sisters came and went, speaking both French and English, laughing often with various relatives and friends and Ronnie's sister, Georgia, and her husband. His sister made great egg and cheese sandwiches.

Everyone was kidding around. I tried to play along, but the drive down to Latchford each day was gut-wrenching. My breathing would be quickened on the drive. As on other painful trips with Ronnie, I had to consciously take deep breaths to maintain my calm and professional demeanor. I had no way to remain detached with people who were now family. Even if Hayley had not grown up with this family, when you see people several times a week in the face of pain and a terminal illness, when everyone is in pyjamas when you visit, when the grandkids are teasing you on the phone, when you are greeted with Fudgsicles, how can this not hurt?

After the three-hour drive to Sudbury, the staff checked him out and found another spot in his neck, where the tumour had spread into his spinal cord. He was given rounds of radiation to his lower spine, as well as his neck. Nicky phoned me at midnight. "I'm at the hospital. I'm so tired. I don't want him to die. I need to be with him. He's so scared. He keeps crying. He's afraid he will never walk again. Can I go back to the motel? I need to sleep but I am afraid to leave him. Is he going to die tonight?"

How could I answer this? I wanted to say, *What the hell do I know?*

"I think he'll be okay. You have to rest. You need to sleep. Go on, call me tomorrow. I will see you in a couple of days when you guys come home."

When Ronnie came home, he had less pain, but he was still unable to walk. "I'm going to get physio, and then I'll be able to walk. Chris will help me get ready," he told me.

Nicky caught my eye. As she walked me out to the car, she spoke quietly, "He isn't going to walk again, is he? Physio won't do much. He gets so tired. But he needs to dream about being able to walk again. I know he's never going to walk again no matter how much physio he gets or how much Chris works to exercise his legs. But we have to keep giving him hope."

The next week, Ronnie's kids and a neighbour got him up into the truck, which was tough because he had been paralyzed since the cancer had eaten into his spine. The family piled cushions around him, and he rode in the back like a prince, with his granddaughter giggling beside him. That old truck barrelled along the Red Squirrel Road with dust flying around it, even though Chris was driving slowly so Ronnie wouldn't bounce around too much. Halfway down the road, Chris slowed right down. Ahead was a bull moose, coming just to say hi to Ronnie. This was a fine farewell for nature to give him.

Ronnie was tired when he got back, and for the next few days he pretty much stayed in bed. But he was excited about the moose. "Right there on the road! It was just waiting for me! Oh, if I had my gun, and the season was still open, he would have been mine. But it was great to just see him."

A few days later Ronnie started to breathe shallowly, irregularly. I wouldn't say much when I was there, unless the family asked me questions in the front yard, out of earshot of Ronnie. When we were with the family and near Ronnie, we kept it light and talked about fishing.

I had delayed taking any time off, but I was scheduled to go to a conference on global health in Ottawa. I overlapped with my locum, Dr. Tim. I brought him over to the Paiges' to meet Ronnie and the family. Tim is tall, tanned, and athletic. He reminds me of my brother. I told him Ronnie needed daily house calls.

All week in Ottawa, I expected a call telling me that Ronnie had passed away. But I came home to find everyone cheerful. Ronnie was alert and laughing. Dr. Tim had visited him every day. He had repositioned the catheter, changed the antibiotic, and read the Bible to Ronnie and his family. Ronnie was a Protestant; he and Nicky had seldom gone to church as she was Catholic. But Ronnie's grandfather had read Ronnie the Bible when he was a boy, and Ronnie found it comforting. The delirium had cleared, and Ronnie was now breathing normally. "It's a miracle!" said Nicky, smiling.

Some days Ronnie would only eat for Chris. Nicky would make him his favourites, like steak frites. Not even a bite. But for Chris, he would eat a half sandwich. Ronnie's daughter, Steph, would try not to meet my eyes, lest she read what was in them. When the family was around Ronnie, we pretended he was going to get well. He had not finalized his will. There was no DNR (Do Not Resuscitate) order on the fridge, the usual place they are kept to guide paramedics who come urgently to dying patients. How could I help Ronnie prepare for death when he was so busy being alive?

One tough day, when Ronnie was not eating and couldn't get out of bed, I asked everyone to leave. There were often several adults gathered around, kids joking, oblivious to the hospital bed in the middle of the living room from where Ronnie presided over his kingdom with a tired smile on his face. It was a bright Indian summer day.

I examined Ronnie and could feel his greatly swollen liver, full of cancer. "You know, Ronnie," I said, "it has been a year since they said your cancer was incurable. It has spread. We're running out of options.

Radiation to the bones was just for pain relief. Chemo, surgery, and radiation have bought you ten years. We can keep switching up your antibiotics. We can keep your pain controlled and your bowels moving. But Ronnie, and it's too hard to say this, it may be days, or even weeks, but you are dying."

"Yeah, that's okay. Can you get Chris in here?"

Chris went in and spoke to Ronnie for a few minutes. He came back out through the French door to the porch and down the ramp that had been installed to accommodate Ronnie's wheelchair. On the front lawn, we spoke in whispers. Chris said, "He wants me to look after Nicky."

That same day I had to slow down as I was driving home on the way into Cobalt, the highway lined with dark pines. Just ahead was a large black brown bear. Was this the kind you run from, or stand still? Definitely, stay in the car. The bear lumbered slowly across the road and disappeared into the bush. The next day Ronnie was out in his wheelchair, supervising as the family butchered a bear in the front yard. Ronnie was still in charge, telling Chris the best way to cut the meat and portion the pieces to be taken to the butcher to be made into sausages or steaks. I loved that Ronnie had a starring role right up to the end. His family kept building on his abilities. His spirit was strong to the end.

Ronnie slept a lot for the next few days. He was just tired right out. He was barely fifty, and he was dying. The following week I was at the clinic. "Hey, come here!" called my secretary, Carla. "Look at Ronnie!" She was gesturing out the window to the street. The whole family was walking past us, Chris pushing Ronnie in his wheelchair, Nicky at his side. His daughter-in-law, Angela, had baby Ronnie in a stroller, and Ronnie's granddaughter Jerzee skipped merrily beside them. Everyone greeted Ronnie as they passed, and he grinned at them; people were so happy to see him out.

That weekend there was a special concert at the Legion, across the street from Ronnie's home. An English guitar player was spending a few days with friends in Latchford. I knew I would be down at Ronnie's anyway, so I figured I could grab a few dances between visits. The musician even had a cover for a song made famous by our friend Eddy's band, "You to Me Are Everything."

I checked on Ronnie, who was pretty much sleeping all the time now, visited with the family, and brought Nicky over to the Legion for one drink. Everyone was happy to see her. The whole community had been dropping in, bringing pies, buns, soup, helping to fix the roof or to move Ronnie. It was great to whirl around the dance floor and try to forget the man who could no longer dance, the one dying in the house across the street. We brought Nicky home, and she began her nightly ritual of moving her bed right up close to Ronnie's, so she could hold him as he slept beside her, comforting him with the warmth of her body.

Thanksgiving Friday I went over to the Paiges' house after clinic. Ronnie's breathing was characterized by Cheyne-Stokes and he was very jaundiced. I had my student, Jen, with me. I think it's important for medical students to see patients at home, to see how much strength family and community can provide, and to see the limits of medicine. Nicky and I shared knowing looks. Ronnie was not really conscious. Most of Nicky's sisters were there. I checked Ronnie's vitals. I knew I was saying goodbye and could barely meet Nicky's eyes. "You have my number. Call if you need me."

The call came around noon on Thanksgiving Monday. Ronnie had just peacefully passed away. I grabbed a tourtière and an apple pie from my freezer and drove back to Latchford. The minister was there, saying prayers with the family. I went over to Ronnie's body and formally listened to his heart with my stethoscope and felt for the absent pulse. I touched his cheek with the back of my hand. I reached over to Nicky. "I am so sorry." I wiped the tears away from my eyes and we hugged. As I made my way through the house, down the ramp, and through the yard to my car, I hugged Nicky's kids, her sisters, Ronnie's sister, Georgia, and their mom, Dorothy. Several kids were playing and laughing; a couple were crying.

Once I got home, I sat in my backyard in the sun reading a mindless murder mystery and listening to what sounded like a thousand birds in the mountain ash and chokecherry trees. Only two apples remained in my three trees, the rest turned into chutney and pies. I had ignored the plums. A few late geese flew overhead. Though I could barely see them, I could hear their mournful cries. How could they see to fly? How do we see to live?

Late that night I went out into my backyard to look at the mysteries of the night sky, the Milky Way with its billions of stars, the few constellations I can still remember. I remembered one late night in early fall, a couple of weeks earlier, when I had paddled my kayak under those stars down at Mowat's Landing, on the Montreal River, with my locum, Dr. Tim, and worried the whole time that Ronnie would die and I would miss the call. I felt that life and death are just too unbearably, breathtakingly full. I had to keep catching my breath.

Ronnie's funeral was a few days later. I had to practise twenty or more times what I would say about this joyous man who died at fifty-two. Even on the way to the Latchford Arena from Haileybury, I wept as I said the words aloud, alone in the car. "Instead of mourning Ronnie, we can live what he has taught us. Every time we help a troubled kid. Every time we fully appreciate the beauty of our Northern Ontario home and its wildlife. When we help a friend in need to fix a roof or a motor. He lived for all of this, and we can help keep his spirit alive when we live this way, too."

The arena was cool, and a drizzly rain came down; we could hear it pattering on the roof. The displays of flowers featured outdoor themes — fishing poles, hunting caps, moose, ducks, and birchbark filled the ceramic vases. Ronnie's ashes had been placed in an urn adorned with a moose. The honour guard who carried that urn away from the arena were Ronnie's grandsons and nephews, some of the many young people Ronnie had inspired. All were wearing hunting caps and camouflage jackets.

At the Legion, we celebrated his life. Nicky set his ashes on the bar and joked with the barmaid, "I sure wouldn't have left him alone with you tending bar when he was alive!"

I had managed not to cry when I spoke at the funeral, but Nicky's brave strength and humour had completely undone me. I wept all the way home.

～ 16 ～

GIFT GIVING

In my practice in Latchford were several couples who had been married for close to fifty years. I found it quite grounding to see two people who remained happy together for such a long time, living and laughing and supporting each other.

Carole and Juergen were one of these couples. Both had salt-and-pepper hair. He was German and spoke with an accent; she was from Timmins. I loved the way they were always smiling at each other. He never complained about his arthritis or diabetes, and she was always cheerful in spite of the different cancers she'd beaten. "I'm just terrific! You should see me skating with my grandchildren!" They smiled as they left the clinic on Monday, holding hands. "We'll get that blood work you want done later today," Carole called over her shoulder.

The following day was a very wintry one, and having ignored the closed highways, I drove slowly to work. It is peaceful in its own way to be alone on the road, the blowing snow around the car, the howling winds, and the feeling that you might be the last person left on Earth, the landscape so eerily devoid of people.

When I got to the clinic, my secretary called out to me, "All the patients have cancelled. Maybe you can just check the labs to make sure there's nothing urgent? I think we should leave soon as the storm is supposed to get worse. There was another accident south of Temagami."

I went into my little office, so cheerful with its mosaic tile desk and stained-glass Tiffany lamp. The computer was already on, so I quickly scrolled through the electronically filed lab values till I came to Carole's. She only had one kidney, and the kidney function value I was reading was shockingly high. For some reason, that one kidney was shutting down.

I immediately grabbed a portable phone and called Carole at home. "Carole, this is Dr. Roedde. How are you? I'm just checking some labs."

"I'm not sure. For some reason, I haven't peed since yesterday. My hands and feet are swollen, and I feel kind of headachy."

"Okay, Carole, I know the roads are closed, even in town. But you have to get to hospital. Right now. Something is wrong with your remaining kidney. I'm going to fax a note to emerg. Is Juergen okay to drive you in this weather?"

"Sure, you know my husband. He's game for anything. We should be there in about fifteen minutes."

I quickly drafted a note to fax to the hospital. *Previous malignant melanoma, in remission. Previous kidney cancer, resected, stable. Elevated kidney function tests of unknown cause. Assess and transfer urgently to urology in Sudbury or admit locally as needed.*

The next day I was teaching third-year medical students. One had been working in emerg when Carole came in, and he filled me in. Carole's creatinine and potassium had continued to climb. An elevated potassium level can cause cardiac arrest. The roads were closed, and the air ambulance also couldn't fly due to fog, so the paramedics had taken her to Sudbury by road. She was hooked up to a drip containing a fancy cocktail of insulin, bicarb, and glucose to bring down the potassium levels, and she was wearing a Ventolin mask. I'd never heard of using Ventolin to bring down potassium. By the time the ambulance arrived in Sudbury four and a half hours later, Carole's creatinine was over one thousand. Normal is around one hundred (creatinine levels are an important indicator of renal health).

CT imaging had shown a non-cancerous mass in her lower back blocking her ureter, causing her one remaining kidney to back up with

171

fluid so she couldn't pee. Emergency urologic surgery put in a stent, bypassing the blockage.

Carole was reflective later, once she'd transferred home. "I think I would have died if you hadn't gone down to the clinic to check those labs, if everyone hadn't acted so quickly. Such a team effort. Juergen driving me to the hospital, you, the emerg staff, the paramedics, the specialist team in Sudbury. All in a Northern Ontario winter, with closed highways for over a day. Life here can be harsh, but we sure can all pull together to make the right things happen. What a gift."

———

Monica's hair was soft and fluffy and spread out like a halo from her head. She was always smiling, though she seldom heard much of what I was saying. She was elegant and liked wearing floral-print blouses with coordinating solid slacks. As I came into the room, her face leaned toward her husband. Monica was eighty-nine years old, and her husband of fifty-six years, Cecil, was eight years her junior. With her head cocked a little to the side, she said, "I'm a little hard of hearing. But Cecil hears for me." His freckled face with its sandy hair was turned toward her.

Monica was a new patient to me but had already experienced nearly nine decades of a lively, engaged life. She smiled at her steady companion — as always, he had her list of meds up to date and knew exactly what was happening in terms of her next appointment for wound care for an infected toe, a complication of her diabetes and poor circulation. He didn't mind getting up at five in the morning every couple of weeks to drive her to the wound clinic in North Bay. "He has always been so good to me!" she would boast. "And before that, he looked after both my parents. My mother had Parkinson's. He helped her in and out of the bath. He looked after my father before that, till he died. I am so lucky to have found a man like this." Cecil would smile and say quietly, "I don't know what I would have done without her. My family threw me out. None of them speak to me after all these years, except my sister Yolanda."

My medical student Adam was with me. I was trying to explain that Monica might lose her toe if it stayed infected. "Your circulation isn't great," I told her. "With the diabetes, it's hard for you to heal. There's a risk the infection will go into the bone. So we might have to take your toe off." I looked over at Adam and nodded, my mouth set tightly.

Monica looked at my third finger and reached over with her worn hand to grasp my ring. "That is lovely." I looked down. A round piece of abalone was surrounded by an oval of filigreed silver. I had bought it in Nepal. I loved that ring.

I took it off and found one bare finger of hers and slid it on. It just fit.

"I love it. Oh, Dr. Roedde, thank you!" She beamed.

The next week, I had a note from Monica. She thanked me for the ring and joked about how the surgeon in North Bay had not offered her his watch, though she had admired it. She praised the skill of the surgeon who'd amputated her toe and also Adam, the medical student she had met with me, who was now working with the surgeon. "Such a nice young man," she said. "He's staying with his parents in North Bay. It was nice to see a familiar face, your student, when I was so scared. I didn't feel any pain." She wrote the note in a flowing, neat, carefully slanted script, her words full of life and warmth.

I saw Cecil and Monica at home as her toe was healing. On one visit, Cecil patted my hand. "Here, I have something for you." He brought over a small wooden shelf with scrollwork, cut-outs of birds and flowers. "I make these. I love doing these designs. Maybe you can put it up in your office?"

Three weeks later, my phone rang just as I was waking up on Sunday morning.

"Hi, Gretchen. It's Stacy Desilets. I'm in the E.R. Your patient Monica Shaw has come in. She isn't doing well. She's not conscious. She doesn't have long."

Immediately, I threw on clothes and drove the ten minutes to the hospital. I spoke quickly with Stacey, who was swamped with patients, then went into Monica's room in the E.R. She was on oxygen. Cecil was there, and he explained to me what had happened. "It was a hard night.

She was short of breath. I called an ambulance early this morning. She slipped as we loaded her into the ambulance. Will you stay with her? I'm exhausted, haven't slept all night. I have to eat something to get some strength."

When Cecil left, I held Monica's hand as she was moved from her E.R. bed to a stretcher, then brought to a private room on the floor. The nurse took out the airway from her mouth. "She will be more comfortable with just the oxygen."

I spoke to her steadily the entire time. The hearing is the last to go, and a dying patient does hear us. I held her hand. The oxygen hissed slightly. I watched her breathing, which was getting more ragged. Then there were long pauses. Her skin was mottling. Her earlobes turned inward. There were more long pauses in her breathing. She sort of shrugged her shoulders — a fancy name for this is decerebrate posturing, which happens when the brain is starting to shut down. Her irregular breathing was another sign. I kept holding her hand and started to say the Lord's Prayer.

"… as we forgive those who trespass against us."

A very long pause. Longer. No breath at all. I pushed the bell. The nurse answered, "Yes?"

"Can you come in? With a stethoscope?"

Doris, the head nurse, came in and listened to Monica's heart — not beating. Up to the neck — no sign of a pulse. "She's gone," she said. "Nine forty a.m. You'll need to take her rings off. I'll bring you some lotion. Where is her husband?"

"He's gone for some breakfast. I'll stay with her."

I kept holding her hand. I looked at this still body. *Where has that life gone?* I kept thinking of Gary Potts from Bear Island telling us that the Ojibwe word for the Creator meant mystery. I held her cooling fingers, with their rings. Doris came back with some lotion and looked over at me. "Thanks for being here with her."

I smoothed the lotion over Monica's fingers and tried to move her rings over her knuckles. On her ring finger were her wedding and engagement rings, locked together with a small catch to hold the loose rings secure. I kept my face still. No tears were in my eyes. I was a doctor in the hospital, armed and defended.

Cecil came quietly into the room.

"She's gone," I told him. "It was peaceful."

Cecil came and held her hands. He lifted one and kissed it. I held her other hand. Together we worked the lotion into her fingers and smoothed off an opal ring. Then a small gold band. Then the one I had given her. I held it in my hand, remembering giving it to her.

Cecil turned to me and said sadly, "What will I do? We would have been married fifty-six years this fall. She's been my best friend for over half a century. She took me in after my family had thrown me out." He held her wedding rings. "Help me get these off. I will treasure them. She loved her jewellery so much. But she would want you to have your ring back. Take it. Keep it and think of her."

One night I woke, troubled, in the middle of the night and could not get back to sleep. Like Monica, I have a collection of jewellery from around the world. So, I puttered around at three in the morning, looking at my own collection. In a jewellery box, I found an antique silver necklace pendant, with a round abalone shell centred in a rectangle with a filigree border. I had never worn it. It matched the abalone shell and filigree silver in the ring I had given to Monica.

The next day on my way home from work I popped into an Indigenous craft shop in Cobalt and bought abalone earrings. For the last few weeks, I've been wearing the silver and shell memories. I am reminded of the last moments in the life of a beautiful woman. The earrings and necklace represented new memories yet to be made. These are linked together, loss and renewal. Alone at home, I could finally weep.

A few weeks later, I ordered some blood work on Cecil. He had no symptoms but was being monitored by our local urologist because of a cancer that was in remission. All the tests had been good at each annual screening, so I was shocked to get the results of the latest test. He had cancer again, and it was spreading rapidly — a different cancer. How could this have happened? We'd been following him so closely. How could I have missed this? Was I so preoccupied with his wife and her illnesses that I had not been alert to Cecil, her caregiver? I phoned him and tried to stay calm as I explained that I was "ordering some extra tests, a bone scan, and an MRI of the pelvis."

When he came in the next week for the results, I tried to speak, but instead I started to cry. I apologized for not being detached about the results as I informed him he had stage 4 cancer that had spread to the bones. He reached over and hugged me, "You are just a sweetheart," he said. "I thought it might be news like this. See, I've brought you more gifts. Here's another piece of scrollwork, a wooden box carved with flowers for the Kleenex box in your office, and a small sign for your desk that says 'Survivor,' because I know you're a cancer survivor, too. I have a wooden mobile as well for Carla's kids. Don't you take her present! I'll give you the number of my sister. For when it's time. So you have someone to call. This is going to be a big disappointment for a few widows who've been trying to talk me into taking holidays with them!" He laughed, gave me another quick hug, and left the office with more strength and dignity than I could ever imagine.

It is such a gift to be blessed with closeness to people such as these.

∽ 17 ᶜ

SWEETGRASS

At the end of the year, December 30, 2014, Mae Katt, Alec's god-mother, came through town with her family. We shared a luncheon feast along with Alec and his family. It turns out that Mae also knew Hayley, Alec's wife, and her family when they were growing up in Latchford. We talked a lot about Mae's mom, Little Mary, who had just passed away. We talked as well about Mae's work helping entire northern communities get off narcotics, using a replacement drug called suboxone to alleviate the withdrawal symptoms. This important work had been highlighted in an Al Jazeera documentary, *Ring of Fire*, which we have watched on YouTube.

As I was unable to go to Bear Island for Little Mary's funeral, I loaded up hampers of food for Mae to take along.

I had just had that year's students from the Northern Ontario School of Medicine for supper: turkey with all the trimmings. I had shown them photos from the 1970s, from the times I was working at Bear Island and flying into the communities in Sioux Lookout Zone. I talked to them about my current patients, several of whom had suffered frostbite when their woodstoves went out. Some who cannot afford electricity heat with wood, and sometimes the fire goes out. It is great to have students who intend to follow those same paths, who plan to work in remote Indigenous communities or low-income non-Indigenous ones — to learn from the people and to teach them.

Two of the pictures showed early motherhood. In the first, I bathed my baby in a round metal tub. In the second, she was wrapped in a blanket and held to my chest as I drove the open steel boat. Where does the time go? How could this infant be the young woman who works as a researcher translating French missionary journals for land claims? She can work from anywhere, and having outgrown Ontario, she has moved to Vancouver — like salmon going back to the spawning grounds, as both sides of her family are from the West.

When she moved out West, Anna brought with her a pair of antique lace-up black boots that had been passed down through the family and given to her by my Aunt Lorraine. Anna presented these to the Roedde House Museum in Vancouver, located in a house that had once belonged to my great-grandfather. Anna lives just a couple of blocks away. The cycle renews, the Medicine Wheel does keep turning, and we are all on it, struggling for meaning.

I thought of the many students who had joined me on house calls, whose insights had enriched my own work. Julia had literally saved one patient's life, helping me to not give up on him as he kept "falling off the wagon" in his shack in Cobalt, and now he was the proud leader in the local AA group while living in a subsidized apartment in Haileybury.

At the time of writing, Alec and his family still live up north, around the corner from me in Haileybury. They moved into the home where Anna used to live. Hayley's son, Regan, is a great artist. A framed print of his that I have on my wall at home is a crazy mix of blues, images of birds and trees and flowers, and a poem by Emily Dickinson about hope. I remember when Alec asked me to bring him sweetgrass for smudging their new home, to bless his new family.

I smiled as I remembered their wedding. It was a crisp blue late summer day in 2013. Family and friends were waiting at the water's edge in Temagami. Bright bouquets of flowers lifted our hearts. The food for the wedding feast to follow was giving off wonderful, rich aromas. Alec stood with his groomsmen, waiting for Hayley, her dad, and her son. We were seated, but Alec stood patiently. Minutes and more minutes passed, and I tried not to look at my watch with worry. Then down the drive, twenty minutes late, came the old, dark green 1947 truck, slowly carrying forward the beautiful bride, her son, Regan, and her dad, Don, who gave her away.

Gary Potts caught my eye and later explained, "I was sending Alec messages of hope. Sometimes you just have to wait. It's not passive, waiting. You can wait actively, hoping, preparing. For this or that hardship to pass. For that truck to start! You let the waiting fill you with strength."

We both laughed.

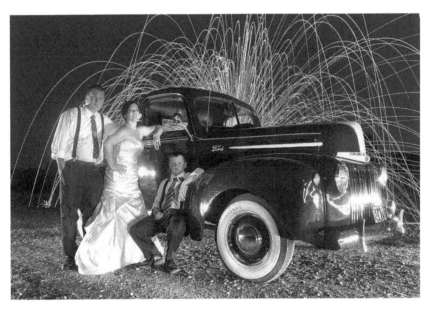

Alec and Hayley, with Regan, on their wedding day, Lake Temagami, August 17, 2013.

∽ 18 ⌒

WINTER WISDOM

The last few geese were flying overhead. It was October 2015. Several of the local men were wearing T-shirts that said, "This marriage has been interrupted by the hunting season!" Plans were being made to go to the "Moose Dance," which celebrates the end of the hunting season and involves a lot of drinking, dancing, and the wearing of fake antlers. My daughter-in-law was out at the hunt camp with Alec and Regan, hoping to get a moose on her due date. My granddaughter, Etta Mae, arrived a week later, delivered at home by the midwives. Eight pounds, nine ounces! Alec was there, with Hayley's mom and sister, and Nicky had brought thirteen-year-old Regan home from the hunt camp. He gave me a big hug when I arrived a few minutes after the birth, tears in his eyes: "I have a new sister!"

A month earlier the same midwives had delivered another Amish child in my home, on a dark night during a thirty-three-hour power failure. We'd carried solar lights, headlamps, and camping lanterns between the labouring and birthing rooms and watched the flashes of sheet lightning across Lake Temiskaming.

One week after my grand-daughter Etta Mae was born, the hunting group got a nearly sixteen-hundred-pound moose, out the Red Squirrel Road. Alec and Hayley got their share — sixty pounds of moose meat for their freezer.

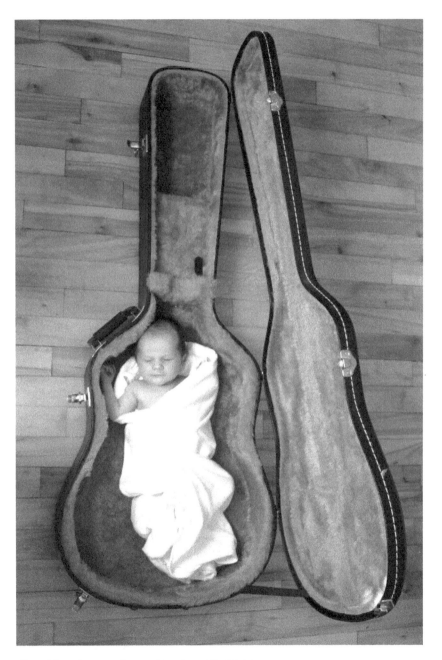

Etta Mae, born at home October 17, 2015.

While Chris, Ronnie's son, was out hunting, he saw a white owl overhead. "Guess that means my grandpa has died." Sure enough, when he called home, Nicky told him that Ronnie's dad had passed. And I remembered Gary Potts telling me about his son Guy dying. "I was at home on Bear Island. Then all the birds just stopped singing. I knew then Guy had passed over. I went outside. I felt my son's spirit. Then a loud chorus of birds started to sing again, and I knew Guy was with me."

Vicki came up to visit Alec's family and see the new baby. "I've been knitting something, but it isn't finished yet. I brought them a dream catcher." It was good to see her. We sat and chatted around my kitchen table in the home overlooking Lake Temiskaming, just as we had sat and chatted many a time on island 762, in Lake Temagami. "Sonny Boy just passed away," explained Vicki. "He had told us he wanted a normal funeral. None of that burning sweetgrass stuff. A Roman Catholic funeral. He was down at the nursing home and asked the staff to get him ready. They asked if he was going out for lunch. 'Yes,' he told them. 'They'll be picking me up.' The nurse shaved him and got him dressed in his best suit, wondering who he was expecting. And then he sat down and died. He knew the spirits were coming to get him. He was buried in that suit."

Alec and his family have had a few musical evenings down at my place. The new baby, Etta Mae, is just a few weeks old, but she already giggles and loves it when I carry her around while I dance to the music, or when I rock her in the bentwood rocker that the Amish community made for me, a thank you for the use of my home. Anna came for a few days, too. We had lively meals and played music long into the night. Alec has noted Etta Mae's long fingers: "Maybe she'll play keyboards!" I watch the musicians and play a couple of songs myself, autoharp or the new guitar. Regan plays guitar and Alec plays anything we have. Hayley and I sing. I am reminded of the many times when my own children were small and live music filled this same living room.

Hayley and I smile. "Big wheel keeps on turning," our voices sing together.

⁓ Acknowledgements ⌒

I would like to thank my family, who has shared this journey with me. I am grateful to my patients and their families, to the health care workers at all levels, and to my students, who work together to support the living, the dying, and those being born. I have been fortunate to have many writing mentors: Karen Connelly, who's guided me through this process; Helen Pereira, my mother, who died in February 2018 a published author in her own right; Bill Roedde, my father, who travelled the world and shared his journeys with us and in print; and my brother, Steve, who lives an amazing life including rowing the Atlantic but lets others tell the tale. The support of the Ontario Arts Council is also gratefully acknowledged. I am particularly thankful to have been welcomed into other communities among the First Nations, the Amish, and Franco-Ontarians, and I accept full responsibility for any errors of cultural misinterpretation. It is a great privilege to be allowed to share the intimate moments of birth, life, and death, and I hope this memoir honours that trust.

᭖ Credits ᭖

IMAGE CREDITS
Bea Shawanda: 30, 31
Danny Turcotte, Catch-Light Photography: 179
Gretchen Roedde: 24, 46, 49, 57, 66, 97, 98, 99, 100, 103, 116, 126
Hayley McKeever: 181

BOOK CREDITS
Developmental Editor: Allison Hirst
Project Editor: Elena Radic
Copy Editor: Robyn So
Proofreader: Tara Tovell

Cover Designer: Laura Boyle
Interior Designer: B.J. Weckerle

Publicist: Elham Ali

DUNDURN
Publisher: J. Kirk Howard
Vice-President: Carl A. Brand
Editorial Director: Kathryn Lane
Artistic Director: Laura Boyle
Production Manager: Rudi Garcia
Director of Sales and Marketing: Synora Van Drine
Publicity Manager: Michelle Melski
Manager, Accounting and Technical Services: Livio Copetti

Editorial: Allison Hirst, Dominic Farrell, Jenny McWha,
Rachel Spence, Elena Radic, Melissa Kawaguchi
Marketing and Publicity: Kendra Martin, Kathryn Bassett,
Elham Ali, Tabassum Siddiqui, Heather McLeod
Design and Production: Sophie Paas-Lang